Health Information Science

With the development of database systems and networking technologies, Hospital Information Management Systems (HIMS) and web-based clinical or medical systems (such as the Medical Director, a generic GP clinical system) are widely used in health and clinical practices. Healthcare and medical service are more data-intensive and evidence-based since electronic health records are now used to track individuals' and communities' health information. These highlights substantially motivate and advance the emergence and the progress of health informatics research and practice. Health Informatics continues to gain interest from both academia and health industries. The significant initiatives of using information, knowledge and communication technologies in health industries ensures patient safety, improve population health and facilitate the delivery of government healthcare services. Books in the series will reflect technology's cross-disciplinary research in IT and health/medical science to assist in disease diagnoses, treatment, prediction and monitoring through the modeling, design, development, visualization, integration and management of health related information. These technologies include information systems, web technologies, data mining, image processing, user interaction and interfaces, sensors and wireless networking, and are applicable to a wide range of health-related information such as medical data, biomedical data, bioinformatics data, and public health data.Series Editor: Yanchun Zhang, Victoria University, Australia Editorial Board: Riccardo Bellazzi, University of Pavia, Italy Leonard Goldschmidt, Stanford University Medical School, USA Frank Hsu, Fordham University, USA Guangyan Huang, Victoria University, Australia Frank Klawonn, Helmholtz Centre for Infection Research, Germany Jiming Liu, Hong Kong Baptist University, Hong Kong, China Zhijun Liu, Hebei University of Engineering, China Gang Luo, University of Utah, USA Jianhua Ma, Hosei University, Japan Vincent Tseng, National Cheng Kung University, Taiwan Dana Zhang, Google, USA Fengfeng Zhou, Shenzhen Institutes of Advanced Technology, Chinese Academy of Sciences, China

More information about this series at http://www.springer.com/series/11944

Li Tao • Jiming Liu

Healthcare Service Management

A Data-Driven Systems Approach

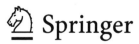 Springer

Li Tao
Southwest University
Beibei
Chong Qing, China

Jiming Liu (iD)
Hong Kong Baptist University
Kowloon, Hong Kong

ISSN 2366-0988   ISSN 2366-0996   (electronic)
Health Information Science
ISBN 978-3-030-15383-0   ISBN 978-3-030-15385-4   (eBook)
https://doi.org/10.1007/978-3-030-15385-4

Library of Congress Control Number: 2019935166

This Springer imprint is published by the registered company Springer Nature Switzerland AG.
The registered company address is: Gewerbestrasse 11, 6330 Cham, Switzerland

Contents

List of Abbreviations

ABM	Agent-based modeling
AOC	Autonomy-Oriented Computing
AOC-CSS	Autonomy-Oriented Computing-based cardiac surgery service
ASIC	Application specific integrated circuits
BNS	Bumped non-urgent surgery
CABG	Coronary artery bypass graft
CCN	Cardiac Care Network of Ontario
CPSO	College of Physicians and Surgeons of Ontario
CS-OR	Cardiac surgery operating rooms
CU	Catheterization unit
D^2CSM	Data-driven complex systems modeling
DSP	Digital signal processors
EHR	Electronic health records
EMR	Electronic medical records
EMW	Median wait times for elective patients
FPGA	Field programmable gate arrays
GIS	Geographical information system
GP	General practitioner
HDASS	Healthcare Decision Analytics and Support System
HHSC	Hamilton Health Science Centre
HIS	Hospital information system
HITS	Hyperlink-induced topic search
HIV	Human immunodeficiency virus
ICES	Institute for Clinical Evaluative Sciences
iHDS	Intelligent healthcare decision support
IMS	Information Management System
KL	Kullback-Leibler
LHIN	Local Health Integration Network
LV	Latent variable
MIS	Management information systems
MOHLTC	Ministry of Health and Long-Term Care

MSMQ-EC	Multi-server multi-queue with an entrance control
MV	Measurement variable
NE	North East
OPHRDC	Ontario Physician Human Resources Data Center
OR	Operating room
PCA	Principle component analysis
PLS	Partial least squares
RI	Recent immigrant
SD	Standard deviation
SEM	Structural equation modeling
SMW	Median wait times for semi-urgent patients
SU	Cardiac surgery unit
TC	Toronto Central
UMW	Median wait times for urgent patients
UUB	Unused urgent time block

List of Figures

List of Tables

Chapter 1
Introduction

A healthcare service system, sometimes also called a health system, a health care system, or a healthcare system, is a system, including people, institutions, and resources, that delivers health care services to promote the public health and wellness of people [1, p. 2]. Like other social systems, a healthcare service system also includes its inputs, such as patient and service resources; its output, such as treated patients and the service performance representing the quality and quantity of provided services; and internal service providers, such as hospitals, clinics, and units. Unlike other simple or complicated systems, patients and service providers (all are referred to as "entities" in this book) in a healthcare service system are autonomous in that they make decisions on their own based on their distinct profiles and a variety of interrelated factors. As a result, entities are self-organized in many cases and may exhibit totally different behaviors, even if they face the same problems and the same affecting factors. Entities may interact with each other through service providing or receiving behavior, or through information sharing. Such interactions may result in feedback loops between entities and impact factors in many cases. Partially due to this reason, a healthcare service system may exhibit certain complex phenomena, such as periodically emptying the queue for specific services [2, p. 47], which may result in unreasonable service performance that is quite different from managers' expectations. Due to the complex nature of a healthcare service system, we are facing challenges in addressing many healthcare service management problems, such as discovering key factors and their effects on wait times, predicting wait times for a specific service in the future, proposing strategies for shortening wait times, and figuring out the underlying reasons that account for the specific spatio-temporal patterns of wait times.

In this chapter, we first introduce a conceptual model for a healthcare service system. We review its complex nature and the importance of the interactions between the factors and entities in the system. Then, we summarize the commonly-faced healthcare service management problems in practice by examining wait time management as an example. We use a data-driven complex systems modeling

© Springer Nature Switzerland AG 2019
L. Tao, J. Liu, *Healthcare Service Management*, Health Information Science,
https://doi.org/10.1007/978-3-030-15385-4_1

(D^2CSM) approach to address problems in wait time management. This approach enables us to systematically understand healthcare services and address the wait time management problems either individually or integratedly using the following four specific methods, i.e., *Structural Equation Modeling (SEM)-based analysis, integrated prediction, service management strategy design and evaluation,* and *behavior-based autonomy-oriented modeling.* We finally present the profiles of the cardiac care system in Ontario, Canada, which is the research scenario in this book.

1.1 Complex Healthcare Service Systems

1.1.1 A Conceptualization of Healthcare Service Systems

According to the open systems theory [3, pp. 149–150] [4, pp. 23–30], a healthcare service system can be normally represented by a conceptual model, as shown in Fig. 1.1. According to this model, a healthcare service system is divided into three parts: (1) multiple service providers that deliver healthcare services (such as hospitals) and are located in different cities or regions; (2) the system's inputs, including patients receiving services and healthcare service resources; and (3) the system's outputs, which involve multiple indicators representing the service performance, such as treated patients and wait times.

A healthcare service system can be divided hierarchically into subsystems or entities at different levels (as shown in Fig. 1.1[1]). For instance, a collection of hospitals in a region can be thought of as a healthcare service system, where each hospital can be viewed as a sub-system or a specific entity. Each sub-system can be further divided into sub-subsystems, which are units consisting of distinct personnel and facilities providing different services to patients. In the real world, the profiles of service providers differ in terms of the number and types of personnel [6, p. 9], such as physicians and general practitioners (GPs); on-site facilities, such as operating rooms (ORs) and laboratories [7]; and costs and financing. Service providers also vary in their service management behavior, such as scheduling time blocks in ORs [8, 9] and referring patients to other service providers [10, 11]. Normally, service providers' profiles and their service management behavior, which are often referred to as healthcare service systems' supply factors [12], determine the actual delivery of services to patients to a significant extent, and thus directly affect the variations of the systems' outputs.

A major input to a healthcare service system is patients. Patients residing in different regions may exhibit distinct profiles because they have differences in their ages [13], education levels [14, 15], social networks [16, 17], and other personal characteristics. Patients' profiles not only affect the incidence of disease, but also influence their autonomous service utilization behavior, which directly determines,

---

[1]Note: This figure was adapted from the open systems model [5, p. 90].

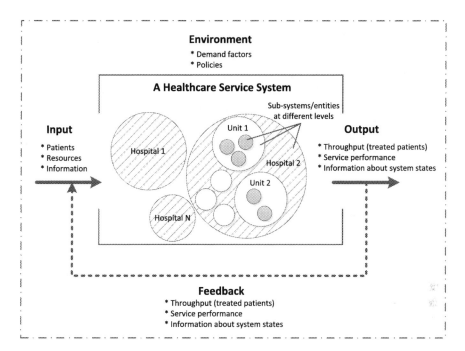

Fig. 1.1 A conceptual model illustrating a complex healthcare service system

to a large extent, the number of patient arrivals at healthcare facilities. Patients' profiles and behavior, called the demand factors [18], may result in patient arrivals varying at different times [19] and in different regions [20]. The inputs of a healthcare service system also include various healthcare service resources, such as newly graduated doctors and nurses, as well as recently purchased medical equipment. These resources are often planned and allocated by healthcare service managers to meet the patients' needs and promote service performance. Another type of input is information. The information input into the system includes various types, such as data about the geodemographic and socioeconomic profiles of a population; people's attitudes towards hospitals, doctors, treatments, and service performance; and even the built and natural environment, like geographic access to services [21, 22], air quality, and seasonal weather [19, 23]. The information normally has different effects on patients' service selection behavior, and hospitals' service management behavior.

The outputs of a healthcare service system mainly include treated patients, service performance, and the relevant information. Service performance is normally represented by various indicators, such as wait times, throughput, in-hospital mortality rate, and re-admission rate. It should be noted that most of the indicators and some of the impact factors are abstract concepts (also called latent variables (LVs) or latent constructs) that should be estimated using several observed variables or measurements. For instance, the wait time indicator can be judged by the median wait times, 90th percentile wait times, or queue length [20, 24], each of which represents one aspect of wait times. Some of the outputs of a healthcare service system will be fed back as inputs of the system. For instance, treated patients may return to a hospital soon after a visit because they get sick again. Patients and hospitals may be aware of the information about the service performance and treatment outcomes in the past. As a result, such feedback information may then affect the behavior of patients when they select healthcare services, or of hospitals when they schedule patients to ORs. Due to the existence of feedback loops, management problems related to a healthcare service system become complex [25–27] and are hard to address.

1.1.2   Complexity and Self-Organizing Nature

As implied in Fig. 1.1, the challenges in addressing healthcare service management problems lies in the complexity and self-organizing nature of a healthcare service system, which include:

1. *Multiple and multi-scale impact factors*: The inputs, outputs, and the behavior of a healthcare service system may be directly or indirectly affected by various factors on different scales, which include, but are not limited to, demographics, socioeconomic backgrounds, and environmental conditions, as well as the healthcare-related behavior of patients [28] and hospitals [29]. For instance, old age (physiological age at a biological scale) is an important risk factor for cardiovascular diseases, while the patient hospital selection behavior at a personal scale may heavily influence the distribution of actual patient flows to various hospitals.
2. *Heterogeneous entities*: Entities can represent system elements, such as patients and physicians, and sub-systems, such as hospitals and units. In a healthcare service system, entities are heterogeneous due to the differences in their profiles and behavior. For instance, patients differ in terms of age, gender, ethnicity, socioeconomic background, lifestyle, decision making style, and their corresponding healthcare service utilization behavior.
3. *Bounded rationality*: In many cases, entities can only access partial information about the system. As a result, as Herbert A. Simon stated [30], entities may have "bounded rationality" and may not exhibit optimal behavior. Patients may select a hospital that had shorter wait times in the past, but now has longer wait times because they do not have access to the latest wait time information about the concerned hospitals.
4. *Interactions and coupling relationships*: Entities may spontaneously interact with multiple impact factors and other entities directly or indirectly. Entities may also be constrained by structural or functional relationships, which are referred to as coupling relationships. The coupling relationships between entities can be either pre-defined or dynamically adjusting. For instance, units in a hospital have coupling relationships with one another due to the functional constraints

of the logistics of patient flows. During the interaction processes, entities exert changes in the environment or in other entities' behavior. As a result, an entity may affect other entities' behavior directly, through their coupling relationships, or indirectly, through the updated environment or through feedback.

5. *Autonomous and adaptive behavior*: Entities in a healthcare service system make decisions and behave rationally based on their own behavioral rules with respect to their perceived environmental information. Their behavior can therefore adapt to a changing environment. For example, in response to regularly released wait time information about each hospital, patients may select different hospitals for specific healthcare services to avoid long wait times.

6. *Emergence and self-organization*: Autonomous entities achieve their goals by adjusting their behavior so as to adapt to the dynamically changing environment and respond to feedback. During this self-organizing process, small changes in variables may cause larger changes in the system under some conditions. As a result, self-organized, spatio-temporal patterns may emerge from the system that are not predefined, indicating that the system is collectively regulated.

Since a healthcare service system is complex and self-organizing, a growing number of studies have attempted to apply complexity science to the study of healthcare service systems. Applying complexity theory to healthcare service systems dates back to the middle of the 1990s, when Priesmeyer et al. used chaos theory, one of the classical complex systems theories [31, 32], to examine clinical pathways as nonlinear and evolving systems. Arndt and Bigelow [33] speculated on the possible applications of chaos and complexity theories for healthcare services management. Begun and White viewed the nursing profession as a complex adaptive system and paid special attention to its inertial patterns [34]. Smethurst and Williams found that the statistical distribution of the variance in wait times to see specialists followed a power-law distribution [35], which indicated that the healthcare service system was self-organizing, possibly due to the interactions between the patients and available doctors. However, to the best of our knowledge, few studies aim to understand a healthcare service system from a self-organizing systems perspective.

1.1.3 Interactions

Interactions play a critical role in the presence of emergence behavior [36] and certain spatio-temporal patterns in a complex system. When one entity interacts with another, or with the environment, information or instructions are exchanged. Here, the interaction refers to a mutual or reciprocal information-exchanging action. In general, there are two types of interactions between entities and between entities and their environment [36]:

- Direct interaction: An entity may directly affect other entities' behavior or states through performing activities or exchanging information. An obvious example is the direct interaction between a doctor and a patient for illness and treatments. Another example suggests that obesity may spread from person to person, especially when people are friends or siblings, because they may exert social influence or peer effects on each other [16]. An entity may also take a direct interaction with its environment via a process of information exchange. For instance, news or advertisements broadcasted by the media in the social environment of a person may cause her to change her health-related behavior [37].

- Indirect interaction: An entity may have effects on other entities' behavior or states indirectly by using the environment as an information-exchanging medium [36]. The indirect interaction process involves two phases. In the first phase, an entity releases information in its environment. Then, in the second phase, other entities will be aware of the information kept in the environment and behave accordingly. The indirect interaction between entities commonly happens in a healthcare service system. For instance, previous studies have suggested that the positive or negative treatment outcome of patients in a hospital may affect the hospital's reputation, which will in turn affect other patients' decisions on selecting the hospital [38]. In this case, patients who are selecting hospitals interact indirectly with the historical patients in the same hospital via the released information about the service outcome.

In some cases, the interactions of the impact factors, especially with autonomous entities' behavior, may form closed causal chains (the so-called "local feedback loops" mentioned in the literature), which can potentially result in unpredictable and/or self-organized behavior of a system. For instance, the long wait times in a hospital may weaken the probability of patients selecting the hospital, which will in turn decrease the number of patient arrivals. Therefore, the wait times in the hospital will be reduced soon afterwards. Furthermore, the interactions and local feedback loops between or among the entities' behavior and impact factors can potentially give rise to certain statistical regularities and spatio-temporal patterns, such as the aforementioned power-law distribution of wait time variations to specialists [39], and the pattern of so-called "oscillatory dynamics" of waiting queues [2, p. 47]. In view of this, it is necessary to model individuals' behavior and interactions to discover the underlying mechanisms that account for the dynamics and emergent patterns of patient arrivals and wait times of healthcare services.

1.2   Practical Healthcare Service Management Problems

Healthcare service management refers to the leadership, process, and general management that provide healthcare services in organizations (e.g., hospitals) [40, p. 78]. Practically speaking, the management, or the administration of healthcare services, usually relates to three aspects [41]:

- Volume and coverage of services, which involve the planning, implementation, and evaluation of services;

- Resources, such as budgets, buildings, equipments, medicines, physicians, nurses, and information;
- External relations and stake holders, which include patients and other users of services.

When managing healthcare services, administrators in different healthcare service systems may find they have several difficult problems in common. We use wait time management for a healthcare service system as an example; the following two scenarios present a few management problems that are commonly faced by healthcare administrators.

Scenario 1

Bob is a hospital administrator at Hamilton Health Science Centre in Ontario. Bob finds that although the hospital has added resources to ORs, the wait times for cardiac surgeries are still too long. He wants to know: (a) What impact factors cause the long waits? (b) How do the impact factors affect the wait times? (c) How can he make a reasonable prediction about patient arrivals in the near future (e.g., the next 5 years) so that the hospital is able to schedule the ORs for shorter wait times?

Scenario 2

Alice is a provincial healthcare administrator in Ontario. She finds that there are some interesting spatio-temporal patterns in patients using healthcare services in the province. She also finds that the current resource allocation method for cardiac surgery services is static, which results in a gap between the estimated and real needs for services in the province. In order to make a reasonable and evidence-based decision on regional resource allocations for cardiac surgeries to shorten the average wait times and reduce disparities in wait times, she wants to know: (a) What causes the spatio-temporal patterns in the patient arrivals and wait times at hospitals in the province? (b) When healthcare resources are allocated in the province, how can she estimate the real needs for each hospital? (c) How can she regulate patient arrivals to hospitals in the province?

In general, the most common management problems for wait times usually relate to the following four closely related issues:

1. *Discovering the effects of certain demand or supply factors on wait times.* Wait times involve multiple demand or supply factors, which may exert direct or indirect effects on patient arrivals and/or wait times. To gain a qualitative understanding of the dynamics of the wait times, we need to figure out how specific factors directly, indirectly, or moderately affect service utilization.
2. *Estimating the changes in wait times with respect to the variations of certain impact factors.* Predicting the changes of wait times in the future is important in formulating effective management strategies. Once the relationships between the demand factors, supply factors, and wait times are identified, it is possible and important to make a prediction of future wait times in accordance with the variations in certain factors.

3. *Designing and evaluating service management strategies for improving wait times.* In addition to the associations between a service provider's profiles and wait times, service management behavior also plays a significant role in service delivery and wait times. We therefore need to design new service management strategies to improve wait times.
4. *Explaining spatio-temporal patterns in wait times.* Patients autonomously decide whether or not to go to a hospital based on specific factors, such as the distance between their home and the hospital, service profiles, and service performance. Patients' autonomous behavior may result in dynamically changing patient arrivals at hospitals, which may then lead to variations in the wait times. Therefore, characterizing the emergent spatio-temporal patterns in wait times could offer crucial insights into the nature of healthcare service systems.

1.2.1   Discovering the Effects of Impact Factors on Wait Times

In reality, the demand and supply impact factors may exert direct, indirect, or moderating effects on wait times. A *direct effect* measures how a dependent variable changes when a predictor variable increases or decreases. A direct effect is commonly represented by a positive or a negative path coefficient (weight) in statistics. For instance, studies have found that the factor of service capacity may directly influence the variations in wait times [29, 42]. Service capacity, therefore, has a direct effect on wait times. An *indirect effect* denotes a predictor variable that influences a dependent variable through a third variable. For instance, the population size imposes an indirect effect on wait times, as a larger population may be translated into a greater number of patient arrivals [43, p. 59], which is one of the direct causes of wait times [44]. A *moderating effect* measures how a third independent variable may change the direction and/or the strength of the relationship between a predictor variable and wait times. For instance, the prevalence of smoking and inactivity, two traditional cardiovascular risk factors, in the less-educated population [14, 19] suggests that a higher proportion of well-educated individuals in the population may mitigate the pressure of population size on patient arrivals, and thus ease the burden on wait times [45]. In this book, the direct, indirect, and moderating effects are referred to as *complex effects*.

From a computational perspective, discovering the direct, indirect, and/or moderating effects of certain demand or supply factors on wait times can be transformed into a research question: How can we explore the complex relationships of predictor variables (e.g., impact factors) with dependent variables (e.g., service utilization and wait times)? Two specific research issues must be addressed to answer this question.

1. *Modeling latent variables (LVs)*: As the concerned variables include those that cannot be directly observed, how can we build a mathematical model to infer an LV from other observed variables?

2. *Modeling complex relationships between variables*: How can we model concurrently direct, indirect, and moderating relationships between the observed
variables and/or LV using mathematical means? How can we quantify these
relationships based on the data?

Existing studies usually rely on multivariate statistical methods to discover the
relationships (i.e., path weights) between the variables from data, such as regression
[46, 47]. These methods often model the relationship between the dependent and
independent variables as a linear, logistic, or other types of functions [48]. However,
these methods have limitations when constructing LVs and modeling the complex
relationships between variables, rather than the pairwise relationships between the
dependent and independent variables.

Therefore, the first objective of this book is *to propose a method to address
the problem of investigating the direct, indirect, and/or moderating relationships
between the observed variables and LVs*.

1.2.2 Estimating the Changes in Wait Times

Estimating the changes in wait times in response to the changes of certain demand
and supply impact factors is, in essence, a problem of estimating the dynamics of
specific dependent variables with respect to the variations in specific predictor variables. Three specific research issues must be addressed to answer this question:

1. *Exploring complex relationships between variables*: Given aggregated data that
describes the dependent and predictor variables of interest, how can we explore
the complex relationships between these variables?
2. *Estimating the changes in specific dependent variables*: Given the trends in the
changes of certain predictor variables, can we obtain the variations in specific
dependent variables in the future based on the identified relationships between
the variables?
3. *Characterizing the dynamics of estimated variables*: As the estimation results
based on variable relationships are somewhat sketchy, how can we determine the
dynamically changing process of focal dependent variables over time?

Existing studies dealing with these research issues in the healthcare context can
be classified into three categories:

1. *Estimations based on pairwise variable relationships*. These studies investigate
the effects of predictors on specific dependent variables using traditional statistical methods, such as regression, which can be used to forecast the changes in
dependent variables if the predictors vary. For instance, the demographic profiles
of population age and ethnicity are two of the most important determinants for
utilizing cardiac surgery services. Cardiovascular risk factors, such as diabetes,
hypertension, and obesity, are higher in the age group of 50 years and above
[13, 19] and vary in different ethnic groups [19, 49]. However, these commonly

used statistical methods may not be able to model LVs and reveal complex relationships between variables.

2. *Forecasts based on specific patterns of variables.* These studies focus on finding the underlying patterns in certain variables, which can then be used to make scenario-based predictions. For example, previous research has found that there are more patient arrivals in the winter compared to other seasons because of the cold weather [19]. The arrivals also vary depending on the time of day and the day of week [50, 51]. Some studies have tried to make forecasts for specific scenarios, such as predicting emergency department arrivals in a disaster [52] or during a pandemic influenza season [53]. However, predictions based on identified patterns require that the scenarios for finding patterns and those for predictions are the same. This requirement is difficult to satisfy in the situation considered in this book, as the scenario may change if specific predictor variables vary.

3. *Predictions based on modeling methods.* These studies attempt to characterize the dynamically changing service performance of a healthcare service system in a given scenario. They usually use queueing models [54] and discrete event simulations [55] to examine the dynamics of service utilization in a healthcare service system and to assess performance variations based on so-called "what-if" studies [54]. However, these studies have not addressed the question of how service performance changes in response to demographic shifts.

Motivated by the above observations, the second objective of this book is *to propose a method for estimating the changes in service utilization and performance in response to the variations of the impact factors.* This method is also required to capture the dynamics of estimated service utilization and service performance over time.

1.2.3   Designing and Evaluating Strategies for Shortening Wait Times

Two specific research questions must be answered in designing and evaluating service management strategies to cope with unpredictable patient arrivals with the goal of making better use of healthcare resources and improving wait times.

1. *Designing strategies*: In view of current healthcare service management strategies and the dynamics of patient arrivals, what new strategies can be proposed?

2. *Evaluating strategies*: With a given scenario describing the patterns of stochastic patient arrivals and the profiles of a specific service provider, how can we model service behavior to provide a test-bed for evaluating the effectiveness of new strategies?

Existing studies have used mathematical methods, such as mathematical programming, to optimize specific measurements to design better service management strategies. The management of time blocks in ORs for cardiac surgery services can be used as an example. One of the most common issues considered when designing new OR time block allocation strategies is how many OR time blocks should be reserved to cope with the unpredictable arrival of urgent patients. Reserving more time blocks than needed can cause decreased OR use, a longer waiting list, and a longer waiting time for non-urgent surgeries. Reserving insufficient time blocks can increase the risk to patients who need urgent care, incur more bumped non-urgent surgeries, and prolong wait times for those bumped cases. To improve the use of OR time blocks, existing studies have used mathematical methods (e.g., job shop scheduling models) to compute the optimal number of reserved urgent time blocks to maximize the use of OR time blocks while minimizing the overtime/cancellation of surgeries [56]. However, these studies have not considered that patient arrivals are dynamic because of the number of impact factors involved, such as the weather and patients' service utilization behavior [19]. Therefore, the theoretical optimal solution may not perform well in an actual healthcare service.

One common way to model service behavior to evaluate different service management strategies is to simulate the service operations with different strategies and to compare the simulated results based on certain measurements. In healthcare service research, the queueing model is commonly used to characterize the behavior of a service provider and examine the dynamics of service performance, such as wait times and queue length. In general, the queueing model describes stochastic patient arrivals and the services delivered by a healthcare service system as a continuous-time or a discrete-time Markov chain, where the system state corresponds to the number of patients in the system. The expected queue lengths and wait times can be mathematically analyzed and the dynamics of service performance can be simulated with a specific queueing method.

The third objective of this book is therefore, *within the context of time block management in ORs, to design an adaptive service management strategy to improve the use of service resources with respect to unpredictable patient arrivals and evaluate the effectiveness of the adaptive strategy in improving service performance.*

1.2.4   Characterizing Spatio-Temporal Patterns in Wait Times

Explaining the spatio-temporal patterns in wait times can be defined as a research question of how to model and simulate individuals' behavior and interactions with respect to certain impact factors, and thus to reveal the underlying mechanisms that account for the observed spatio-temporal patterns in wait times. Three specific issues must be addressed to answer this question:

1. *Modeling entities*: What specific autonomous entities potentially play significant roles in the emergent patterns and thus should be modeled, and how should they be defined within the model?
2. *Modeling entities' behavior, interactions, and local feedback loop(s) with respect to certain factors*: Which behavior of the entities, major impact factors, and

the interactions between them are relevant to the observed spatio-temporal patterns in wait times, and hence should be investigated and modeled? As local feedback loops [57] formed by relationships between the variables may amplify or dampen the effects of factors or entities' behavior on wait times and thus result in nonlinear dynamics in the system, which local feedback loop(s) should be modeled? How can we model entities' behavior and formulate the rules that govern this behavior, while taking into account the identified effects of factors and the heterogeneity of the entities?

3. *Carrying out simulation-based experiments*: What spatio-temporal patterns at a systems level emerge from the simulation? Are the simulated emergent patterns similar to those observed in the real world? If a simulation based on the developed model can reproduce the spatio-temporal patterns observed in the real world, what are the underlying mechanisms that account for the emergent patterns?

Existing studies have used the methods of stochastic modeling and simulations, system dynamics, and agent-based modeling (ABM) to model the behavior of a healthcare service system and simulate the dynamics or spatio-temporal patterns of wait times. We summarize the major characteristics of these methods below:

1. *Stochastic modeling and simulations* aim to model a service system by defining the service profiles, service management behavior, and stochastic properties, such as Poisson arrivals and exponential services. Two classic methods are the queueing model and discrete event simulation. As these methods require that assumptions be made regarding the stochastic properties, they may encounter a number of difficulties in characterizing the spatio-temporal patterns of the wait times. The assumptions about the stochastic properties of a healthcare service system may be strong and not always hold true in the real world. Further, these methods cannot explore how entities' behavior and interactions result in the emergent spatio-temporal patterns at a system level, because they do not aim to model the entities' heterogeneous behavior.

2. *System dynamics* models a focal system as a causal loop diagram [58]. A system dynamics model contains entities (referred to as "stocks" in this method) that accumulate or are exhausted over time, and their interactions (referred to as "flows" in this method) are usually represented by first-order differential or integral equations [59]. Unlike other methods, system dynamics pays special attention to modeling the internal interactions between entities and local feedback loops [57] within a system. However, it is difficult to model the heterogeneous and autonomous behavior of each entity with this model, as it assumes that each entity's behavior is fixed. Therefore, this method cannot explain how entities' behavior and interactions cause the emergent patterns in a healthcare service system.

3. *Agent based modeling* (ABM) [60] attempts to model a healthcare service system by defining agents (i.e., entities), their behavior, and interactions. However, traditional ABM faces a major challenge in characterizing system-level emergent patterns; it lacks the general principles to explicitly indicate which fundamental

behavior of and interactions between agents play crucial roles in the emerging spatio-temporal patterns and therefore should be modeled. Many existing models based on ABM are more or less ad hoc, with a major focus of delicately defining agents, whereas few of them pay attention to explaining the underlying mechanisms for emergent patterns in a healthcare service system.

Based on the above motivations, the fourth objective of this book is *to propose a modeling method to uncover the working mechanisms that account for the emergent patterns in wait times in a specific healthcare service system.*

1.3 A Data-Driven Complex Systems Modeling Approach

In this section, we present a data-driven complex systems modeling approach (D^2CSM) for systematically understanding healthcare services and for addressing the service management issues. Figure 1.2 summarizes the D^2CSM. As shown in the box on the left side of Fig. 1.2, the D^2CSM uses four specific methods, which include *Structural Equation Modeling (SEM)-based analysis, integrated prediction, service management strategy design and evaluation,* and *behavior-based autonomy-oriented modeling,* to address different management problems in a healthcare service system. Specifically, this book uses these methods to unveil the potential reasons for, and the working mechanisms behind, the observed patterns in wait times in a real-world cardiac care system in Ontario, Canada, by taking the wait time management problem as an example (as highlighted in the right-hand-side box of Fig. 1.2). Further details about the D^2CSM are presented below.

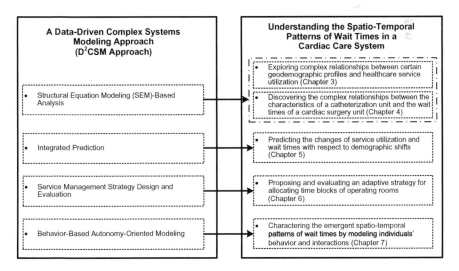

Fig. 1.2 An overall framework of the data-driven complex systems modeling approach

1.3.1 SEM-Based Analysis

To explore the complex relationships between observed variables and latent variables (LVs), we propose the *Structural Equation Modeling (SEM)-based analysis
method* in this book. In general, SEM has the ability to construct LVs [61]
and permits the exploration and confirmation of complex relationships between
variables concurrently [61, 62]. The SEM-based analysis method explicitly includes
four steps:

1. Defining LVs and developing hypotheses related to the direct, indirect, and
   moderating relationships between the observed variables and LVs based on the
   literature;
2. Constructing a conceptual model that contains the complex relationships between
   the observed variables and LVs under consideration;
3. Using SEM to test the hypotheses with data;
4. Interpreting the test results by comparing the discovered relationships between
   variables with those reported in the literature or observed in the real world.

To demonstrate and implement the SEM-based analysis method, we explore the
complex effects of certain demand or supply impact factors on patient arrivals and
wait times in a real-world cardiac care system in Ontario, Canada (this work is
shown in Chaps. 3 and 4). In Chap. 3, the direct and moderating effects of specific
geodemographic profiles (i.e., *population size, age profile, service accessibility,*
and *education profile*) on the *service utilization* of cardiac surgery services are
examined. Based on publicly-available aggregated data on the geodemographic
profiles of Ontario and the corresponding cardiac surgery services between 2004
and 2007, the data test results show that *service accessibility* and *education profile*
alleviate the effects of *population size* and *age profile* on *service utilization*. This
finding reveals that the changes in population profiles due to population growth and
aging may significantly affect the use of cardiac surgery services. It also suggests the
importance of considering the geodemographic profiles of a geographic area and, in
some cases, its neighboring areas, when allocating healthcare service resources, thus
strategically improving service utilization and reducing wait times.

In Chap. 4, the effects of a catheterization unit's (CU's) characteristics (e.g.,
service utilization, capacity, throughput, and *wait times*) on *wait times* in the subsequent cardiac surgery unit (SU) are investigated. Based on published aggregated
data on catheterization and cardiac surgery services, our findings show that *wait
times* in the CU have a direct positive effect on *wait times* in the SU. This is a novel
result, as prior research has seldom examined the influence of one unit's *wait times*
on *wait times* in a subsequent unit in the patient flow process. Our findings also show
that the *service utilization* and *wait times* of a preceding unit are good predictors for
the *wait times* of subsequent units, suggesting that such cross-unit effects must be
considered if the *wait times* in a healthcare service system are to be alleviated.

1.3.2   Integrated Prediction

To predict the wait times with respect to the changes of some impact factors, this book proposes an *integrated prediction* method for estimating the changes in service utilization and performance in response to demographic shifts. Our proposed prediction method consists of three steps:

1. Applying SEM to identify complex relationships between certain impact factors, such as immigration profile, age profile, and healthcare service characteristics (e.g., service utilization, physician supply, OR capacity, throughput, and wait times);
2. Estimating the changes in service utilization and performance using the discovered variable relationships, which are assumed to hold true during the estimation period;
3. Constructing specific queueing models and conducting simulation-based experiments to present the dynamics of the estimated service performance over time.

To demonstrate the implementation of the integrated projection method in solving real world problems, Chap. 5 presents a study that employs this method to estimate the regional use of cardiac surgery services in Ontario between 2010 and 2011, based on statistics between 2005 and 2007. The findings show that our analytical method is able to identify the complex effects of the age profile, recent immigrant profile, and the characteristics of cardiac surgery services on service utilization; describe the variations in service utilization with respect to demographic shifts; and demonstrate the temporal changes in the estimated cardiac surgery performance in terms of the queue length. The work presented in this chapter can enable a healthcare service system to dynamically adjust its resources and management strategies, and thus maintain stable service performance in the face of demographic changes.

1.3.3   Service Management Strategy Design and Evaluation

To design effective service management strategies for the better utilization of healthcare resources and improvement in the service performance, such as the wait times in a complex healthcare service system, it is critical to effectively utilize the feedback information about historical patient arrivals and wait times. In this book, we propose a method to *design and evaluate service management strategies* from a self-organizing systems perspective, with the aim of proposing adaptive service management strategies to improve wait times. In general, this method includes the following three main steps:

1. Determining the feedback related to the managed resources, wait times, and patients, based on which designing adaptive strategies to manage the resources;

2. Developing a queueing model to characterize the patient arrivals and service operations for a specific healthcare service in the real world, which is the testbed for the evaluation of the proposed adaptive strategies;
3. Conducting discrete-event simulations based on the developed queueing model to evaluate the effectiveness of the adaptive strategies in the better use of healthcare resources and shortening wait times as compared to those traditional management strategies;

To demonstrate how to design an adaptive strategy for managing healthcare resources, Chap. 6 shows a study that proposes an adaptive OR time block allocation strategy. This strategy incorporates historical information about OR use when allocating OR time blocks. ORs may thus adaptively schedule their time blocks in response to any unpredictable changes in patient arrivals and hence achieve a trade-off between the number of bumped non-urgent surgeries and any unused urgent time blocks. To evaluate the performance of the proposed adaptive allocation strategy, we developed a multi-priority, multi-server, non-preemptive queueing model with an entrance control mechanism to characterize the general perioperative practice of the cardiac surgery ORs in the Hamilton Health Sciences Centre in Ontario, Canada. By applying the adaptive strategy to this queueing model, we show that our adaptive strategy is able to efficiently regulate the OR time block reservations in response to dynamically changing patient arrivals. This adaptive strategy is able to maintain a better trade-off between the number of bumped non-urgent surgeries and the number of unused urgent OR time blocks, which leads to shorter waiting lists and wait times. Furthermore, our experimental findings suggest that frequently adjusting the OR time block allocation, approximately once a month, helps to improve OR utilization. This finding has the potential to improve the practice of cardiac surgery services.

1.3.4 Behavior-Based Autonomy-Oriented Modeling

In order to model the spatio-temporal patterns of the wait times in a health-care service system, we propose a *behavior-based autonomy-oriented modeling* method based on *Autonomy-Oriented Computing* (AOC) [36]. Autonomy-Oriented Computing [63] is a computational modeling and problem-solving paradigm with a special focus on addressing the issues of self-organization and interactivity by modeling heterogeneous individuals (entities), autonomous behavior, and the mutual interactions between entities and certain impact factors. Compared with agent-based modeling (ABM), AOC is more practical for discovering the underlying mechanisms for self-organized patterns, as AOC provides a general principle, i.e., *AOC-by-prototyping* [64], for explicitly stating what fundamental behavior of and interactions between entities should be modeled. Based on AOC, our pro-posed behavior-based autonomy-oriented modeling method contains the following steps:

1. *Autonomy-oriented modeling*: Modeling entities, environments, entities' behav-ior, behavioral rules, and interactions from a self-organizing systems perspective

based on AOC. This step can be further divided into the following three sub-steps:

- *Identify entities, key impact factors, and local feedback loops*: In the first sub-step, autonomous entities, the key impact factors, the mutual interactions between entities and factors, and the local feedback loops that may play significant roles in the self-organization of the system should be recognized based on the literature and the observations of the system.
- *Identify environmental characteristics and define environment*: In the second sub-step, the types of information that are collected and exchanged in the environment should be determined. Accordingly, the environment that entities reside in and interact with should be formally modeled.
- *Define entities, autonomous behavior, and behavioral rules*: This sub-step handles the modeling and the design of local-autonomy-oriented entities, their autonomous behavior, and behavioral rules. This step needs to clearly state how entities react with respect to different impact factors and respond to various types of information, and how entities directly, or indirectly interact via information sharing, interact with the environment, with a special attention to how the interactions form positive or negative feedback loops.

2. *Simulation-based experiments*: Conducting simulations based on the autonomy-oriented model. During the experiments, the empirical spatio-temporal patterns that are identified from the real world may be utilized to initialize the settings and to parameterize and evaluate the model.

The behavior-based autonomy-oriented modeling method should be an evolutionary and exploratory process to make the synthetic model as real-world driven as possible. During this process, some parameters are initialized and configured to make the synthetic model approximate the real system more closely. The final synthetic model can be used to reveal the underlying mechanisms of positive-feedback-based aggregations or negative-feedback-based regulations, which may account for the observed self-organization and emergent behavior of the real system.

To demonstrate the implementation of the behavior-based autonomy-oriented modeling method in addressing practical problems, Chap. 7 presents a study to uncover the underlying mechanisms for certain spatio-temporal patterns in wait times as observed in the cardiac care system in Ontario, Canada. We developed an Autonomy-Oriented Computing-based cardiac surgery service (AOC-CSS) model to characterize the behavior and interactions of patients and hospitals in cardiac care. We then carried out simulation-based experiments from which spatio-temporal patterns in patient arrivals and wait times emerged. These simulated emergent patterns, especially the statistical power-law distribution of the wait time variations, suggest that patients' hospital selection behavior and its relationship with hospital wait times may account for the self-regulation of the service utilization and wait times. The experiments also revealed that this method can be effective in explaining the self-organized regularities and investigating emergent phenomena in complex healthcare systems.

1.4 Research Context: A Cardiac Care System in Ontario

To better demonstrate the effectiveness of the proposed methods in dealing with the wait time management problems, we chose the cardiac care system in Ontario, Canada, as the research scenario. As shown in Fig. 1.3, 11 Cardiac Care Network of Ontario (CCN)[2] member hospitals that provide cardiac surgery services are unevenly distributed across 14 local health integration networks (LHINs).[3] In Ontario, CCN is a network of 18 member hospitals providing cardiac services in Ontario. LHINs are geographic-location-based, sub-provincial administrative units responsible for determining the healthcare service needs and priorities for their corresponding areas. Their covered geographic areas are shown in Table 1.1. The relationships between the 11 CCN member hospitals and the corresponding LHINs are shown in Table 1.2 [65, p. 20].

LHINs differ from each other in terms of their geodemographic profiles such as population size, age structure, education levels, and immigration. To get the profiles of LHINs, we selected 47 major cities and towns with populations of more than 40,000 according to the 2006 Canadian census.[4] Figure 1.4 (based on Google map[5])

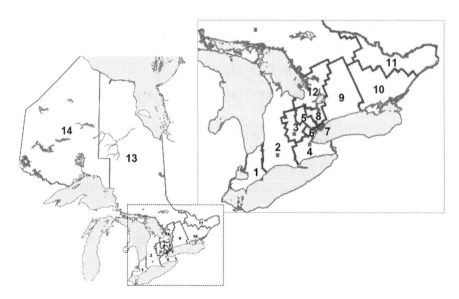

Fig. 1.3 The distribution of hospitals that provide cardiac surgery services across the LHINs in Ontario, Canada. Red dots denote hospital locations and the numbers correspond to the LHIN IDs as shown in Table 1.1

---

[2]https://www.corhealthontario.ca/. Last accessed on April 11, 2019.

[3]http://www.lhins.on.ca/home.aspx. Last accessed on April 11, 2019.

[4]http://www12.statcan.gc.ca/census-recensement/2006/index-eng.cfm. Last accessed on April 10, 2019.

[5]https://maps.google.com/.

Table 1.1 The names, geographical areas, and scopes of LHINs in Ontario, Canada

ID	LHIN name	Area (km^2)	PD	Boundary (Major cities/towns/counties)
1	Erie St. Clair	7323.7	86.1	Windsor, Lambton, Chatham-Kent, and Essex
2	South West	20903.5	43.1	London, Stratford, Elgin, Middlesex, Oxford, Perth, Huron, Bruce, and part of Grey
3	Waterloo Wellington	4746.6	144.6	Wellington, Waterloo, Guelph, and part of Grey
4	Hamilton Niagara Haldimand Brant	6473.0	203.3	Hamilton, Niagara, Haldimand, Brant, and parts of Halton and Norfolk
5	Central West	2590.0	285.7	Dufferin, parts of Peel, York, and Toronto
6	Mississauga Halton	1053.7	956.7	Mississauga, parts of Toronto, Peel, and Halton
7	Toronto Central	192.0	5678.9	A large part of Toronto
8	Central	2730.5	561.3	Parts of Toronto, York, and Simcoe
9	Central East	15274.1	93.8	Durham, Kawartha Lakes, Haliburton, Highlands, Heterborough, parts of Northumberland, and Toronto
10	South East	17887.2	26.1	Kingston, Hastings, Lennox and Addington, Prince Edward, and Frontenac
11	Champlain	1763.1	65.1	Ottawa, Renfrew, Prescott and Russell, Stormont, and Dundas and Glengarry
12	North Simcoe Muskoka	8372.3	50.5	Muskoka, parts of Simcoe and Grey
13	North East	395576.7	1.4	Nipissing, Parry Sound, Sudbury, Algoma, Cochrane, and part of Kenora
14	North West	406819.6	0.6	Thunder Bay, Rainy River, and most of Kenora

PD: population density.

shows the locations of the sampled cities and towns. The 40,000 population cut-off point ensures that the sampled cities and towns represent approximately 90.72% of Ontario's population.

Data about the cardiac care services and LHINs' geodemographic profiles in Ontario are publicly available. In general, two types of aggregated data [66, 67] have been collected and used. The first type of data is *survey data* [67], which is collected and published by government agencies, stakeholders in healthcare, and service providers. Survey data provide information about the profiles and behavior of individuals and service providers. For instance, the Census Bureau provides survey data about the demographics, socioeconomics, and land of a region [68]. Healthcare organizations, such as the Cardiac Care Network of Ontario (CCN) and the Ontario Physician Human Resources Data Center (OPHRDC) have published survey data on patient hospital selection behavior [28] and the number of physicians in each hospital in Ontario by specialty.

Table 1.2 The relationship between the CCN member hospitals that provide cardiac surgery services and the corresponding LHINs

LHIN name	CCN member hospitals
South West	London Health Sciences Centre
Waterloo Wellington	St. Mary's General Hospital
Hamilton Niagara Haldimand Brant	Hamilton Health Sciences
Mississauga Halton	Trillium Health Partners
Toronto Central	St. Michael's Hospital
	University Health Network
	Sunnybrook Health Sciences Centre
Central	Southlake Regional Health Centre
South East	Kingston General Hospital
Champlain	University of Ottawa Heart Institute
North East	Hôpital Régional de Sudbury Regional Hospital

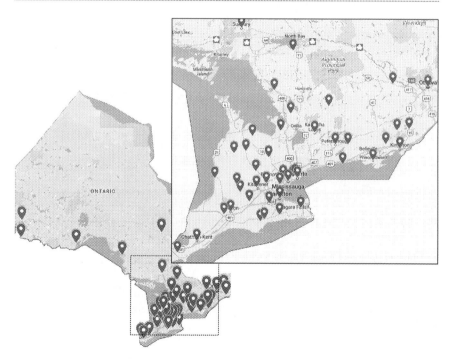

Fig. 1.4 The locations of the sampling cities in Ontario, Canada

The second type of data is *administrative data*, which is often collected by healthcare organizations and service providers "for administrative, regulatory, healthcare operations . . . purposes" [66, p. 73]. Administrative data can represent information about service profiles, behavior, and performance. For instance, the Institute for Clinical Evaluative Sciences (ICES) and the CCN have reported statistical data to

Table 1.3 A summary of the major data sources for the LHINs' geodemographics and cardiac care services that are used in this book

Data types	Data sources	Link
Geodemographics	Statistics Canada: 2006 Census of Population	http://www12.statcan.gc.ca/census-recensement/2006/index-eng.cfm
	Local Health Integration Networks (LHIN)	http://www.lhins.on.ca/home.aspx
	Google Map	https://maps.google.com/
Cardiac Services	Cardiac Care Network of Ontario (CCN)	http://www.ccn.on.ca/ccn_public/FormsHome/HomePage.aspx
	Ontario Physician Human Resources Data Center (OPHRDC)	http://www.ophrdc.org/
	Institute for Clinical Evaluative Sciences (ICES)	https://www.ices.on.ca/
	College of Physicians and Surgeons of Ontario (CPSO)	http://www.cpso.on.ca/
	Ministry of Health and Long-Term Care (MOHLTC)	http://www.health.gov.on.ca/en/
	Auditor General of Ontario Hospitals	http://www.auditor.on.ca/

The last access time for links listed in this table was April 10, 2019.

show the performance of cardiac care services in Ontario in terms of the throughput, median wait times, 90th percentile wait times, and queue length [20, 69]. The College of Physicians and Surgeons of Ontario (CPSO), the governing body for medical doctors in Ontario, provides detailed information about physicians (such as physician name, physician type, and practice locations) for hospitals in each LHIN. The major aggregated data sets that are utilized in this book are summarized in Table 1.3.

1.5 Structure of This Book

This book is organized as follows.

Chapter 2 briefly reviews existing studies and methods for empirically identifying relationships between variables and characterizing the behavior of a healthcare service system.

Chapter 3 presents the use of SEM-based analysis to discover the direct and moderating effects that certain geodemographic profiles exert on service utilization, focusing on cardiac surgery services in Ontario, Canada.

Chapter 4 also demonstrates the effectiveness of the SEM-based analysis, exploring the direct and indirect effects of a CU's characteristics on the wait times of its subsequent SU.

Chapter 5 presents our integrated prediction method for estimating the changes in service utilization and service performance with respect to demographic shifts, within the context of cardiac surgery services in Ontario.

Chapter 6 proposes and evaluates an adaptive OR time block allocation strategy that is designed from a self-organizing systems perspective to cope with unpredictable patient arrivals.

Chapter 7 presents the use of a behavior-based autonomy-oriented modeling method to find underlying working mechanisms that account for certain emergent spatio-temporal patterns in patient arrivals and wait times.

Chapter 8 presents an intelligent healthcare decision support (iHDS) system that incorporates the D^2CSM approach. Two working examples, one for the OR time block allocation, and another for the regional healthcare resource allocation, are also demonstrated to illustrate how our proposed methods and the corresponding iHDS system work for analyzing and supporting healthcare-related decisions.

Chapter 2
Data Analytics and Modeling Methods for Healthcare Service Systems

In order to better utilize healthcare services and improve wait times, we should know what factors cause long waits. How do the factors affect the wait times? How can we estimate the changes in the wait times, taking into account the dynamics of patient arrivals as well as some impact factors? What strategies can be proposed to efficiently utilize healthcare service resources and thus shorten wait times? How can we characterize the dynamics of patient arrivals and wait times? These are common questions that have long been a concern in healthcare systems. This chapter reviews the commonly employed methods to address these questions.

We first present the basic notations and concepts of a healthcare service system. We then examine the commonly used multivariate methods for understanding a healthcare service system by empirically identifying the relationships between the variables. Finally, we survey the modeling and simulation methods that have been used to characterize the behavior of specific healthcare service systems, and unveil the underlying mechanisms that cause the emergent spatio-temporal patterns at a systems level.

2.1 Basic Notations and Concepts

From a systems perspective, a *healthcare service system* (the conceptual model of which is shown in Fig. 1.1) is an open system that exchanges patients, resources, and information with the *environment* [70, p. 32] via its *inputs* and *outputs*. Formally, a healthcare service system S_H can be characterized by a set $S_H = \{R, S, P, X, G\}$, where $R = \{r_1, r_2, \cdots, r_{N_R}\}$ corresponds to the resources within the system, including personnel and facilities, and N_R is the number of dimensions representing the resources; S denotes the organizational structure of these resources; $P = \{p_1, p_2, \cdots, p_{N_P}\}$ represents the *processes*, referred to as the *behavior* of the system, and N_P is the total number of processes that serve patients; X describes

© Springer Nature Switzerland AG 2019

L. Tao, J. Liu, *Healthcare Service Management*, Health Information Science,
https://doi.org/10.1007/978-3-030-15385-4_2

the states of the system at time t, $X = \{x_1(t), x_2(t), \cdots, x_{N_X}(t)\}$, and N_X is the number of dimensions for measuring the states of the system; and G is the goal set of the system.

All of the elements that are outside a healthcare service system and can potentially affect its inputs, structure, and processes are referred to as the environment E of the system, $E = \{e_1(t), e_2(t), \cdots, e_{N_E}(t)\}$, where N_E is the number of elements. The system's environment therefore includes all of the factors that affect the system and are affected by it. A healthcare service system is capable of taking in patients, resources, and information from its environment as inputs, $I = \{i_1(t), i_2(t), \cdots, i_{N_I}(t)\}$, where N_I is the number of different input elements. The system then processes the inputs in some way and returns the treated patients and information about the system states and service performance to its environment as outputs, $O = \{o_1(t), o_2(t), \cdots, o_{N_O}(t)\}$, where N_O is the number of different output elements.

A copy of the outputs may be fed back as part of the inputs into the healthcare service system and may cause changes in the system's transformation processes and/or future outputs. This output information is then referred to as a system feedback F, $F = \{f_1(t), f_2(t), \cdots, f_{N_F}(t)\}$, where N_F is the number of different feedback elements. Feedback can be both positive and negative. Positive feedback tends to reinforce the output of the system, whereas negative feedback regulates it. Feedback can affect the inputs and processes of the healthcare service system at different levels. For example, in response to feedback information about the service performance of each hospital, patients may make different service utilization and hospital selection decisions, and thus influence the inputs to the system, each hospital, and specific units. With the same feedback information, hospitals and units within the system may adjust their processes and/or reallocate their resources to improve the performance of their services in the future.

2.2 Empirical Identification of the Relationships Between Variables

To shed light on what causes changes in wait times, studies on healthcare services have usually used multivariate analysis methods to statistically analyze empirical data to unveil the underlying relationships between variables. In this section, we review the typical types of relationships that healthcare service research has focused on and the multivariate analysis methods that are commonly used to reveal them.

2.2.1   Types of Relationships

Studies on healthcare services have usually identified three types of statistical relationships between different variables, which are referred to as "complex relationships" in this book.

- *Direct relationship*: A direct relationship occurs when a dependent variable (e.g., o_i) is directly affected by an independent predictor variable (e.g., i_i or r_i). This relationship is measured by the direct effect that represents the extent to which the dependent variable changes when the predictor variable increases by 1 unit. Studies have found, for example, that an input variable, service utilization [42, 71], and a resource variable, service capacity [29, 42, 72], are direct predictors of 2 output variables, wait times, and queue length.
- *Indirect relationship*: An indirect relationship exists when an independent variable influences a dependent variable via the effect of a third variable, commonly known as a mediator variable. The indirect effect, which reflects the indirect relationship between the dependent variable (e.g., i_i) and the independent variable (e.g., e_i or r_i), is a product of the direct effect between the independent and the mediator (e.g., e_j or i_j) variables, and that between the mediator and the dependent variables. In the literature, a few indirect relationships between the inputs I and outputs O of the healthcare service system have been identified. For example, a previous study [73] found that the patient satisfaction (an output variable o_i) of the received treatment may mediate the relationship between the service capacity (a resource variable r_i in a S_H) and the behavior of revisiting a hospital (a demand factor should be regarded as an environmental variable e_i as defined in Sect. 1.1.1).
- *Moderating relationship*: A moderating relationship exists when the direction and/or strength of the relationship between two variables (e.g., e_i and i_i) depends on a third variable (e.g., e_j), which is known as a moderator variable. A few studies have discovered moderating effects in healthcare service systems. For instance, a demand factor (also an environmental variable, as defined in Sect. 1.1.1), education, may moderate the relationship between another environmental variable, population size, and an input variable, patient arrivals. This is potentially because the prevalence of smoking and inactivity, two traditional cardiovascular risk factors, in a less-educated population [14, 19] suggests that a higher proportion of well-educated individuals in the population may mitigate the pressure of the population size on patient arrivals [45].

The relationship between two variables can be either linear, meaning that the changes in the dependent variable (e.g., o_i) are proportional to the changes in the independent variable (e.g., e_i or i_i), or nonlinear, indicating that the changes in the dependent variable do not correspond to constant changes in the independent variable. Many researchers have assumed that the variables under consideration are linearly related and thus use linear-model-based statistical methods, such as linear regression, principle component analysis (PCA), and factor analysis, to discover the underlying relationships. Other researchers believe that variables are not only linearly related, and thus employ other nonlinear functions to characterize the more complex underlying relationships, such as using the logistic function to model the resource-limited exponential growth of wait times.

2.2.2 Multivariate Analysis

Three requirements must be satisfied to identify the relationships between variables in a healthcare service system.

1. *Constructing observed and latent variables*: The variables, such as those that affect wait times in a healthcare service system, can be observed or unobserved, as discussed on page 3 in Sect. 1.1.1. The observed variables and latent variables (LVs) must therefore be modeled simultaneously.
2. *Exploring complex relationships between multiple variables*: Variables in a healthcare service system may have direct, indirect, or moderating relationships with each other, which are referred to as *complex relationships* in this book. Thus, we must be able to test complex relationships between multiple variables.
3. *Supporting limited-data analysis*: Publicly available data about a healthcare service system is usually aggregated and limited. We should therefore be able to explore the relationships between multiple variables using limited data.

Existing studies have commonly used PCA [74] to summarize a set of uncorrelated variables from empirical data [75], e.g., to extract the key predictors for wait times. PCA "converts a set of possibly correlated variables into a set of values of linearly uncorrelated variables" called the principal components [75]. PCA is based on the following assumptions: the observed variables are partially correlated; the relationships between all of the observed variables are linear; each pair of observed variables should display a bivariate normal distribution to represent random sampling; and the data describing the observed variables should be metric (interval/ratio) data. PCA may therefore help to transform a set of potentially correlated observed variables, e.g., $\{e_1(t), e_2(t), \cdots, e_{N_E}(t)\}$, into a set of uncorrelated variables, e.g., $\{e'_1(t), e'_2(t), \cdots, e'_{N'_E}(t)\}$, $N'_E \leq N_E$, when analyzing a healthcare service system. For instance, PCA can extract potential key factors in wait times from empirical data on the environment, the input, or the healthcare service system. However, this method cannot reveal complex relationships between variables and cannot model LVs.

Unlike PCA, factor analysis identifies unobserved variables (i.e., LVs), called factors, which can explain the variability between a set of observed and correlated variables. Factor analysis is based on the following assumptions: One or more underlying factors can account for the variation between the given observed variables; variables are partially correlated; each factor is a linear construction of several observed variables; and the data representing the observed variables should be metric data. Factor analysis has been used to extract various underlying factors in healthcare service systems, such as those that contribute to long wait times [76] and patient satisfaction with diabetes care [77]. Factor analysis may help to extract a smaller set of LVs by removing redundancies or duplications from the correlated observed variables. However, it cannot be used to discover different relationships between multiple LVs.

To unveil the relationships between variables from limited data, most studies have relied on multiple regression [46, 47]. Multiple regression is a general statistical method for analyzing the relationship(s) between a dependent and multiple independent variables [48]. This method consists of several types of techniques that model relationships using different linear or nonlinear equations. Studies have usually used multiple linear regression to estimate the contributions of different predictor variables (e.g., e_i, i_i, and r_i) to wait times, assuming that these variables are linearly related. For instance, researchers have used this method to explore the direct effects of hospitals' characteristics (e.g., a university/regional hospital or a county/district county hospital) and patient socioeconomic profiles on wait times [78]. One study used multiple linear regression to examine whether old age (≥ 65) affects wait times in emergency departments [46]. However, this method identifies pairwise relationships between observed variables, and thus is not appropriate for modeling LVs or discovering indirect and moderating relationships between variables.

Some studies in healthcare have used logistic regression to deal with research questions, like whether and to what extent environmental variable e_i, input variable i_i, and/or system resources variable r_i can predict long wait times. Logistic regression is a special type of regression that assumes that the logit of the observed dependent variable is a linear function of the observed independent variables [79]. Studies have used logistic regression to investigate, for example, whether patients under 65 years old and with a lower level of education are more likely to report unacceptable wait times [47], and whether the distance from the homes of Canadian children with cancer to oncology treatment centers has a significant effect on wait times in the corresponding services [80]. Nevertheless, as the aim of logistic regression is to identify a logistic relationship between an observed dependent variable and one or more observed independent variable(s), this method cannot construct LVs or uncover complex relationships between variables.

In the past decade, a so-called second-generation statistical technique, structural equation modeling (SEM), has garnered attention. SEM enables us to simultaneously investigate a series of direct, indirect, and moderating relationships between observed variables and LVs [48]. SEM uses a measurement model and a structural model to discover the complex relationships between variables. The measurement model [48] characterizes the linear relationships between the observed variables (i.e., measurement variables, MVs) and the corresponding LVs. One of the typical ways to relate MVs to LVs is through the reflective measurement model, in which each LV is reflected in its corresponding MV. The structural model [48] describes the linear relationships between LVs. There are two classes of SEM: Partial least squares (PLS)-based SEM and covariance-based SEM [61]. PLS-based SEM is more suitable for theory building and allows for both confirmatory and exploratory modeling, while covariance-based SEM is more suitable for theory testing and is more efficient for confirmatory modeling [61]. Due to the advantages of SEM, healthcare service studies have used SEM to test a "patient satisfaction theory" in emergency departments [81] and to investigate whether depressive symptoms are associated with glycemic control in diabetic adults and the extent to which these adults' health behavior can explain the association [82]. SEM was applicable in our study for analyzing the direct, indirect, and moderating relationships between MVs and LVs of the environment E, inputs I, healthcare service system S_H, and outputs O.

Based on the identified relationships between variables, healthcare administrators can predict the variations in the input or output variables if certain determinants change. The assumption for making predictions based on variable relationships is that the relationships do not change from the baseline period to the prediction period. For instance, studies have used regression models to estimate the future costs of care for cardiovascular disease from 2010 to 2030 in the United States [83], predict the mental health costs in the United Kingdom [84], and estimate the medical expenditures, healthcare use, and mortality in Switzerland in 2010 based on the data in 2009 [85]. However, regression methods may not capture the indirect and moderating relationships between variables, which may influence the accuracy of the predictions in the studies that rely on these models. These predictions also cannot demonstrate how the predicted variables change over time.

Some studies have made predictions based on time series data using the autocorrelation method. Autocorrelation describes the correlation of a random time series with itself at different time delays [86, p. 459]. It makes linear predictions based on the assumption that the observed time series is self-similar. Autocorrelation has been used, for instance, to assess the burden of children suffering from severe viral respiratory illness in an intensive care unit [87]. However, autocorrelation cannot describe the dynamics of a system's behavior.

2.3   Characterization of System Behavior

Studies that use multivariate analysis methods are able to empirically identify the statistical relationships between multiple variables in a healthcare service system. However, these studies cannot deal with the problem of how and why the statistical relationships are formed in a system. To address this problem, we should model and simulate the behavior of a healthcare service system to satisfy the following two requirements.

1. *Modeling heterogeneous and autonomous entities*: In a healthcare service system, entities (e.g., patients and hospitals) are shown in heterogeneity profiles and behave autonomously based their own decisions. Thus, any modeling method should consider how to model the heterogeneous and autonomous entities.
2. *Incorporating interactions*: In a healthcare service system, the mutual interactions between variables and entities at different levels potentially cause positive-feedback-based aggregations and nonlinear dynamics. Any modeling method should therefore incorporate the interaction issue.

To gain an understanding of the dynamics of the wait times, studies have commonly used stochastic modeling and simulation, system dynamics, and agent-based modeling (ABM) to model and simulate the behavior of a healthcare service system. In this section, we review these methods, their advantages, and the challenges in using them to characterize specific spatio-temporal patterns at a systems level. We discuss Autonomy-Oriented Computing (AOC), a research paradigm that is effective in modeling and addressing self-organization issues in complex systems, and thus may help us uncover the mechanisms that account for the spatio-temporal patterns in wait times.

2.3.1   Stochastic Modeling and Simulation

In the delivery of healthcare services, patient arrivals and services to patients exhibit a variability. The input of patients may dynamically change over time because of unpredictable outbreaks of specific diseases and patients' autonomous behavior. Hassan et al. empirically validated the common use of the Poisson distribution to describe stochastic patient arrivals based on the recorded data on patient arrivals in 2000 [88]. The time required for serving patients varies from one patient to another, due to the differences in patients' conditions and the severity of their illnesses. The majority of studies have described stochastic services using an exponential distribution [89].

Studies have used stochastic modeling and simulation methods to model a healthcare service system by describing the stochastic input I and the processes P that transform I to the output O of a healthcare service system. The aim of these methods is to estimate the probability distributions of potential outputs or states, taking into account random variations in one or more variables in the system. Queueing theory (and the corresponding queueing models) is a method in this category that analyzes queue lengths and wait times in a system over time [54].

The origin of queueing theory may date back to the work of A.K. Erlang in the beginning of the last century [90]. Models based on queueing theory are able to mathematically analyze queue lengths and wait times in a system by specifying its random patient arrivals, random delivering services, on-site servers, and scheduling strategies. Models built using queueing theory make the following assumptions: random variables in a system statistically follow specific distributions, e.g., Poisson arrivals and an exponential service rate; entities in the queues are passive, meaning that they cannot make autonomous decisions and interact with each other; and the system state, which is characterized by the lengths of the queues, satisfies a Markov property (i.e., the future state of the system is conditional on the present state of the system, but does not rely on the past state) [91]. Based on these assumptions, this method uses a Markov chain with a transition rate matrix on a state space to describe a system.

Theoretically, we can calculate the steady-state distributions of a modeled healthcare service system with a specific queueing model and thus obtain the system's expected queue lengths and wait times. Here, the steady-state indicates a state of equilibrium in which the distribution properties of a healthcare service system are independent of time [92]. However, in some cases, it may be difficult to use equations to describe the randomness and interdependence of certain random variables (e.g., patient arrivals and wait times), due to the coupling relationships and mutual interactions between these variables. In some complicated queueing models, it may also be difficult to mathematically analyze the steady-state distributions of the modeled system.

To address this problem, studies have used the method of discrete event simulation, which originated around 1960 [93], to simulate queueing models. This method portrays a system's states as a discrete sequence of events [94, 95]. An event may present a specific action (e.g., a patient joins a service waiting queue), which causes a change in the system's state. Discrete event simulation is quite different from the continuous simulation that is suited for systems with continuously changing variables.

To simulate a healthcare service system's random inputs of patient arrivals and its processes, discrete event simulations usually integrate the Monte Carlo simulation. Discrete event simulations are often used to model deterministic systems, whereas Monte Carlo simulations sample a new value for each random variable from specific statistical distributions. Thus, a Monte Carlo simulation can effectively simulate healthcare service systems in which probability and non-determinism play a major role.

Stochastic modeling and simulation methods, especially queueing theory and discrete-event simulation, lend themselves to the analysis and prediction of the dynamic behavior of a healthcare service system. For instance, researchers used queueing models and discrete event simulations to analyze waiting lists for operating rooms (ORs) and recovery rooms under the constraint of the capacity (e.g., beds and recovery time) [42, 96], and to predict the performance of a healthcare service system in different scenarios [54]. Jun et al. in 1999 [97], Fone et al. in 2003 [98], and Jacobson et al. in 2006 [55] surveyed the application of queueing models and discrete-event simulations in the healthcare service literature in addressing problems, such as forecasting the dynamics of patient flows with different resource allocation strategies. In 2010, Günal et al. [99] and Cardoen et al. [100] further reviewed the latest studies that used these two methods for OR planning, scheduling, and performance modeling.

Despite the widespread application of stochastic modeling and simulation methods in healthcare, the statistical assumptions made for the stochastic properties are relatively strong and do not always hold true in the real world. Further, these methods assume the existence of passive entities in the system, thereby making it difficult to model entities' autonomous behavior with respect to certain impact factors. Therefore, these methods cannot be used to explain how spatio-temporal patterns in wait times emerge from individuals' behavior and interactions.

2.3.2 System Dynamics

System dynamics is another commonly used method for modeling and simulating healthcare service systems. It originated in the 1950s [101] and is promoted by the System Dynamics Society.[1] System dynamics is used to explain the dynamically changing behavior of a complex system by defining the interactions (which are referred to as "flows") between variables (which are referred to as "stocks") that may accumulate or be exhausted over time [59]. Stochastic modeling and simulation methods characterize a healthcare service system by describing its stochastic properties, whereas system dynamics uses a causal loop diagram to model the internal feedback loops between the variables within a system. System dynamics assumes that the focal system is deterministic and can be described by a set of coupled, linear or nonlinear, first-order differential or integral equations. In addition, it also assumes that entities contained in a stock are homogeneous, and that interactions between variables, i.e., flows, are predefined and do not change.

System dynamics has been applied to modeling a variety of healthcare services. For example, it has been used to qualitatively characterize the effects of interrelated impact factors and wait times on the cardiac care system in Ontario, Canada [65]. It also has been employed to model the relationships between multiple interacting diseases, healthcare service systems for delivering corresponding services, and national and state policy [102]. Furthermore, it has been utilized to identify bottlenecks in emergency healthcare by simulating patient flows [103], and to predict the demand for ambulatory healthcare services [104].

Due to its advantages in understanding the behavior of a system by modeling stocks, flows, and internal feedback loops, system dynamics provides a potentially useful means for us to investigate how the interactions between multiple variables and time delays affect the dynamics of wait times in a healthcare service system. However, system dynamics may not fully fulfill the requirements for explaining the causes of spatio-temporal patterns in wait times. The homogeneity assumption relating to stocks makes it difficult to model patients' heterogeneous behavior, which depends on individuals' profiles, decision-making styles, and environmental information. The predefined, fixed interactions between stocks do not allow system dynamics to model individuals' adaptive and autonomous behavior. Hence, this method cannot be used to investigate how spatio-temporal patterns in wait times at a systems level emerge from individuals' collective behavior and interactions.

---

[1] http://www.systemdynamics.org/. Last accessed on April 11, 2019.

2.3.3 Individual-Based Modeling

Studies in healthcare have also developed various system models based on individual-based modeling methods. Unlike stochastic modeling methods, which focus on characterizing the uncertainty in a healthcare service system, and system dynamics, which focuses on feedback loops and time delays in a deterministic healthcare service system, individual-based modeling methods describe a system by modeling and simulating the behavior of and interactions between autonomous individuals [105]. Agent-based modeling (ABM), which originated from Neumann's cellular automata machine [106] in the 1940s and Conway's Game of Life in 1970 [107], is a traditional individual-based modeling method that is commonly used in healthcare service research.

ABM regards each individual as an agent, which could be either a physical element, such as a patient, or an abstract concept, such as a hospital. In ABM, each agent makes decisions individually according to its behavioral rules and perceived environmental information [108]. Agents can interact with each other through competition, cooperation, or environmental information sharing. Even a simple agent-based model can develop specific spatio-temporal patterns at a systems level, due to autonomy and interactions [109, 110]. ABM therefore enables us to explore the mechanisms that potentially explain how systems behavior and certain spatio-temporal patterns arise from individuals' behavior and the interactions between them.

Developing an agent-based model for characterizing a healthcare service system is challenging, as it requires a thorough understanding of the modeling system which is inherently complex, and there is uncertainty in designing and quantifying individuals' behavior and interactions [111, 112]. Currently, although a unifying framework for designing, constructing, and validating agent-based models is lacking [113, 114], several frameworks [115], or so called "meta-models" [111], have been proposed to guide the agent-based modeling of complex systems. The frameworks are either domain-driven or pattern-orientated.

- *Domain-driven* frameworks begin with identifying and understanding the domain of the system to be modeled. Developers or modelers then build up corresponding agent-based models and conduct simulations based on the domain knowledge and a specific research context. Domain-driven frameworks, such as CoSMoS, which is proposed and promoted by the CoSMoS Project group[2] [116], may eliminate the uncertainties involved in the modeling and simulation of domain-specific systems.
- *Pattern-oriented* frameworks identify multiple patterns of behavior in real systems. The patterns are used to determine the modeling scope and reduce parameter uncertainty in simulations. Pattern-oriented modeling, proposed by

---

[2]http://www.cosmos-research.org/about.html. Last accessed on April 11, 2019.

Grimm et al. [115, 117], is an example and is effective in modeling real systems [118].

ABM also lends itself to understanding healthcare service systems. Researchers have built different agent-based models to examine the effects of physicians' behavior on patient outcomes [119], predict the spread of infectious diseases based on social networks [120, 121], and evaluate patient scheduling or other operation management strategies [122, 123].

Although ABM provides a potentially useful means for characterizing the behavior of a system by modeling individuals' heterogeneous behavior and interactions, it still faces several difficulties in modeling a healthcare service system and explaining its emergent spatio-temporal patterns. As different agents, such as the modeled patients and hospitals, have various types of behavior and interactions in the real world, does ABM need to model the agents' behavior and interactions as explicitly as possible? What fundamental behavior and interactions at an individual level are crucial for emerging spatio-temporal patterns at a systems level and must therefore be modeled? If the model incorporates too many details, it may become too complex to assess the effects of individuals' behavior and interactions, and other variables on the whole system. If the model omits key behavior and/or interactions, it may not capture the complex, self-organizing nature of a healthcare service system. Thus, the modeled system may not show the spatio-temporal patterns at the systems level. Few studies have successfully discovered the underlying mechanisms for the emergent patterns of a healthcare service system using ABM, which may be due to the above reasons.

In this regard, multi-agent Autonomy-Oriented Computing (AOC) [63, p. 9] offers a promising alternative to solving the problems faced by ABM. AOC is a research paradigm that uses autonomous entities (agents) to deal with the issues of modeling and analyzing complex systems, and solving computational problems from a complex systems perspective [36, 64]. The *AOC-by-prototyping* technique [64] can be used to model a complex system from a self-organizing perspective. AOC-by-prototyping requires recognizing and modeling the autonomous entities that may play significant roles in the self-organization of the system; determining and modeling the types of information that are collected and exchanged in the environment; and identifying and modeling the entities' behavior, their direct interactions or indirect interactions via sharing information in the environment, and the positive or negative feedback loops, which may enable the system to exhibit collective aggregations or regulations. AOC-by-prototyping should be a recursively trial-and-error process to make the synthetic system as faithful as possible. During this process, some parameters are initialized and configured to make the synthetic model approximate the real system more closely. The final synthetic model can be used to reveal the underlying mechanisms of positive-feedback-based aggregations andor negative-feedback-based regulations, which may account for the observed self-organization and emergent behavior of the real system.

Due to the advantages of modeling a system from a self-organizing perspective, the effectiveness of AOC has been validated in a variety of real-world applications, such as understanding the dynamics of the interactions between the human immun-odeficiency virus (HIV) and the human immune system [124]. AOC therefore offers a method for developing a specific healthcare service model to characterize the dynamics of and spatio-temporal patterns in wait times.

2.4 Summary

Wait time management is a long-term problem. This chapter first introduced the basic notations of a healthcare service system with its inputs, outputs, environment, and feedback. We then summarized the types of relationships between variables in a healthcare service system and the methods that can be used to empirically identify these relationships from limited data. These methods typically include PCA, factor analysis, multiple regression, logistic regression, and SEM. These methods face the challenge of discovering complex relationships between observed and latent variables. Utilizing the identified relationships between variables, we can further make predictions for wait times in the future, or, estimate future wait times using time-series-based analysis methods, such as autocorrelation. However, these predictions cannot explain why and how the predicted variables change over time. We reviewed the modeling and simulation methods that may be used to characterize the behavior of a system and to simulate the dynamics of wait times. The traditional methods include stochastic modeling and simulation methods, such as queueing theory and discrete event simulation, system dynamics, and individual-based modeling methods such as ABM. However, these methods face different challenges in modeling a healthcare service system to explain its emergent spatio-temporal patterns.

Based on this review, we presented the motivation for developing the *data-driven complex systems modeling approach* that consists of *SEM-based analysis, integrated prediction, service management strategy design and evaluation*, and *behavior-based autonomy-oriented modeling* to understand the nature of a complex healthcare service system in terms of wait times. We also evaluated the differences between the methods used in existing studies and those considered in this book.

Chapter 3
Effects of Demand Factors on Service Utilization

Although the literature has associated demand factors, such as geodemographics, with healthcare service utilization, little is known about how these factors—such as the population size, age profile, service accessibility, and educational profile—interact to influence service utilization, and thus indirectly affect wait times. Figure 3.1a presents the research focus of how this problem fits into the context of understanding a healthcare service system. Using the Structural Equation Modeling (SEM)-based analysis method to address this problem, we first discuss our research hypotheses and propose a conceptual model based on a thorough literature review. Then, we evaluate these hypotheses using the results of SEM on real world data. Figure 3.1b summarizes the main steps of SEM-based analysis.

This chapter presents an example that employs the SEM-based analysis method to explore whether certain demand factors, i.e., *population size*, *age profile*, *service accessibility*, and *educational profile*, have direct or moderating effects on *service utilization* in cardiac care services in Ontario, Canada. The example in this chapter provides a qualitative illustration of the effects of some geodemographics profiles on the dynamics of patient arrivals and on the changes in the wait times.

3.1 Introduction

Geodemographic factors, such as population size [43], age [13, 125], geographic accessibility to services [22], and level of education [126, 127], have been recognized as important determinants of healthcare service utilization [128, 129]. Geodemographic factors are conventionally used to estimate healthcare needs (e.g., the population needs-based funding formula [130]) to develop better resource allocation and shorter wait times. The majority of studies have focused on examining pair-wise relationships between geodemographic factors and healthcare service

© Springer Nature Switzerland AG 2019
L. Tao, J. Liu, *Healthcare Service Management*, Health Information Science,
https://doi.org/10.1007/978-3-030-15385-4_3

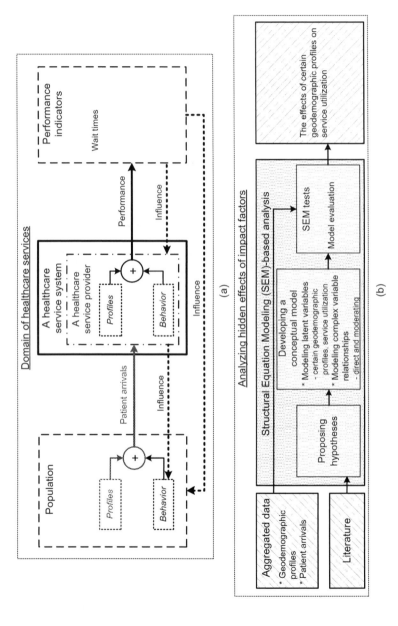

Fig. 3.1 A schematic diagram illustrating the use of SEM-based analysis to explore the complex effects of certain geodemographic profiles on healthcare service utilization. (**a**) The research focus of this chapter (highlighted in red) with respect to the larger context of understanding a healthcare service system. (**b**) The research steps of the SEM-based analysis method in this chapter

utilization, with a scarcity of research exploring how the geodemographic factors interact to affect healthcare service utilization.

Nevertheless, as previous studies have suggested [14, 22, 131], certain geodemographic factors may moderate (i.e., change the direction and/or strength of) [48] the effects that other geodemographic factors have on healthcare service utilization. For instance, if one area has more healthcare service providers, the burden of population growth and aging on the patient arrivals for a specific hospital in that area may be alleviated, as patients residing there have more choices and thus will be more likely to be distributed among multiple hospitals. Geographic accessibility to services (referred to hereafter as service accessibility) [22] may therefore have moderating effects on the relationships between a population's size, age profile, and service utilization. As an additional example, individuals, including seniors, with different education backgrounds may have different lifestyles [14] that can influence their risk for cardiovascular disease [126, 127] and their healthcare service utilization behavior [131]. The educational profile may therefore have a moderating effect on the relationship between population size and healthcare service utilization.

In view of this, in this chapter, we employ the Structural Equation Modeling (SEM)-based analysis to examine both the direct and moderating effects of geodemographic profiles on service utilization within the context of cardiac care, in various sub-regions of Ontario, Canada. The sub-regions of concern are Local Health Integration Network (LHINs) as introduced in Sect. 1.4. Although LHINs have been in operation for years, there is a lack of academic research examining how their geodemographic profiles affect healthcare service utilization.

Following the research steps of using SEM-based analysis method to examine the direct and moderating effects of geodemographic profiles, we firstly develop hypotheses based on the literature review and construct a corresponding conceptual model. We then test the model using SEM [48, 61], based on publicly available aggregated data representing the geodemographic factors and cardiac surgery service utilization in Ontario from 2004 to 2007.

3.2 The Effects of Geodemographic Profiles

According to the literature, the geodemographic factors considered in the work presented in this chapter include the population size, age profile, service accessibility, educational profile. In this section, we review the literature and develop hypotheses regarding the effects of geodemographic profiles (as direct antecedents and moderators) on healthcare service utilization.

3.2.1 Hypotheses

3.2.1.1 The Direct Effect of *Population Size* on *Service Utilization*

Population size, representing the total population that may use the cardiac surgery services in an LHIN, has been shown to exert a direct positive influence on *service utilization*, which is represented by the number of patient arrivals. A larger population may translate into a greater number of people using healthcare services to prevent or treat various types of illnesses [43, p. 59]. Population growth, which can produce more cardiovascular patients, has been identified as one of the major driving forces behind changes in the number of patient arrivals [65]. We thus hypothesize that:

Hypothesis 1 (H1) *Population size* has a direct positive effect on *service utilization*.

3.2.1.2 The Direct Effect of *Age Profile* on *Service Utilization*

Age profile, here defined as the proportion of seniors (i.e., those older than 50) in the population that may use the cardiac surgery services in an LHIN, has been recognized as another important factor that may influence service utilization. Old age is a traditional cardiovascular risk factor [132]. Other risk factors for cardiovascular disease, such as hypertension, obesity, and physical inactivity, are also more prevalent in the segment of the population aged 50 and above [133, 134]. Further, age groups vary in their healthcare service utilization behavior [13, 125], with seniors typically exhibiting a higher rate of use. A larger senior population may therefore result in more cardiovascular patients [135], leading to a greater number of patient arrivals for healthcare services, such as cardiac surgery [65]. Therefore, we hypothesize that:

Hypothesis 2 (H2) *Age profile* has a direct positive effect on *service utilization*.

3.2.1.3 The Moderating Effects of *Service Accessibility*

Geographic accessibility to healthcare services in an area (i.e., *service accessibility*) is an important factor influencing patients' decisions regarding the use of such services [21, 22, 28]. Seidel et al. [21] found that patients' willingness to use healthcare services was negatively associated with the distance between their residences and the destination hospital. A survey conducted by the Cardiac Care Network of Ontario (CCN) [28] showed that the driving distance between home and a hospital was one of the most important factors for patients in choosing a specific hospital, and that more than 80% of cardiovascular patients were not willing to visit hospitals far from home. Extending these findings, we conjecture that if there are several accessible hospitals in one area, patient arrivals for any one particular hospital may decrease, as the difference in the time needed for patients to travel to one hospital or another is negligible. Under such circumstances, we would expect patients to be dispersed among several hospitals, resulting in reduced wait times at any particular hospital in the area.

In this study, higher service accessibility for an LHIN implies that residents in that LHIN have access to more possible healthcare service providers. As a result, the number of patient arrivals at any one hospital in the LHIN may decrease. The pressure of population size or the age profile on each of the hospitals in an LHIN with higher service accessibility may be mitigated, because patients (including seniors) in that LHIN are likely to be dispersed among several hospitals. Thus we hypothesize that:

Hypothesis 3.1 (H3.1) *Service accessibility* has a direct negative effect on *service utilization.*

Hypothesis 3.2 (H3.2) *Service accessibility* has a negative moderating effect on the relationship between the *population size* and *service utilization.*

Hypothesis 3.3 (H3.3) *Service accessibility* has a negative moderating effect on the relationship between the *age profile* and *service utilization.*

3.2.1.4   The Moderating Effects of *Educational Profile*

Educational profile is defined as the proportion of well-educated individuals (i.e., those with more than a high school education) in the population that may use the cardiac surgery services in an LHIN and is an important factor that may also affect healthcare service utilization. Individuals with different education backgrounds manifest different lifestyles [14] and are thus associated with different levels of risk for cardiovascular disease [126, 127] and different service utilization behavior [131]. For instance, a longitudinal secondary data study in Canada showed that smoking and inactivity, two traditional cardiovascular risk factors, were more prevalent in the less well-educated (senior) population [14]. This study suggested that people in the less well-educated group might have a higher demand for healthcare services related to cardiovascular disease. Another study showed that diabetic patients who were at greater risk for cardiovascular disease were more willing to perform self-care behavior if they were well-educated [131]. These findings suggest that, in addition to directly affecting service utilization, a higher proportion of well-educated individuals in the population may mitigate the pressure of population size and aging on service utilization. Thus, we hypothesize that:

Hypothesis 4.1 (H4.1) *Educational profile* has a direct negative effect on *service utilization.*

Hypothesis 4.2 (H4.2) *Educational profile* has a negative moderating effect on the relationship between *population size* and *service utilization.*

Hypothesis 4.3 (H4.3) *Educational profile* has a negative moderating effect on the relationship between *age profile* and *service utilization.*

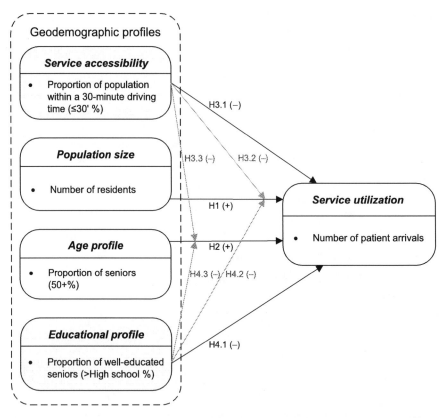

Fig. 3.2 A conceptual model for exploring the effects of geodemographic profiles on service utilization. +/−: a positive/negative relationship between two LVs

3.2.2   The Conceptual Model

The research model, presented in Fig. 3.2, illustrates the hypothesized relationships to be tested in this chapter.

3.3   SEM Tests and Results

3.3.1   Aggregated Data

Within the context of Cardiac Care in Ontario as introduced in Sect. 1.4, we use corresponding aggregated data from 2004 to 2007 to test the hypothesized relationships. Specifically, LHINs' geodemographic profiles with respect to *population size*, *age profile*, and *educational profile* derive from the 47 sampled cities and towns (as shown in Fig. 1.4) based on the Canadian census data. According to the census data released by Statistics Canada, the geodemographic changes from year to year in each LHIN are rather gradual. For instance, between the 2001 and 2006 censuses, the population in Ontario grew by approximately 6.6% [68]. Thus, it is reasonable to assume that the 2006 Canadian census data will approximately reflect the geodemographics of Ontario between 2004 and 2007.

Patients residing in an LHIN may travel to other LHINs to receive cardiac surgeries. For example, 25% of patients residing in the Central West LHIN received treatments from hospitals in the Mississauga Halton LHIN in the 2007/2008 fiscal year [136]. We therefore estimate the population that could potentially use the cardiac surgery services in each LHIN, including those residents living in other LHINs, and thereafter derive the corresponding geodemographic profiles.

The measurement value for *population size* of LHIN i is calculated by:

$$PS'_i = \sum_{j=1}^{14} PS_j PT_{ji} \quad (i, j \in [1, 14], i \neq j), \tag{3.1}$$

where PS'_i denotes the measurement value of *population size* in LHIN i, PS_j represents the population size in LHIN j, and PT_{ji} is the proportion of patients residing in LHIN j but receiving services in LHIN i. The data representing PT_{ji} were obtained from [136].

The measurement values for *age profile* and *educational profile* for LHIN i are calculated by:

$$V'_i = \frac{\sum_{j=1}^{14} V_j PT_{ji}}{PS'_i} \quad (i, j \in [1, 14], i \neq j), \tag{3.2}$$

where V'_i denotes either the proportion of the senior/well-educated population in LHIN i; V_j denotes the number of people aged 50 and above, or the number of well-educated people in LHIN j, respectively.

We operationalize *service accessibility* as the proportion of the population residing within a 30-min driving time to the nearest hospitals providing cardiac surgery services in an LHIN [137]. The 30-min driving time is selected as a threshold to measure healthcare service accessibility in accordance with previous work [138, 139] and the CCN's recommendations [140]. The driving time from each selected city or town to the nearest hospital that provides cardiac surgery services is estimated using the "Get directions" function in Google Maps. In Google Maps, a city or town is represented by the central point of its polygonal area.[1] Unlike a geographical information system (GIS), which estimates driving time based on the lengths of roads and road speed limits [141, 142], Google Maps considers the actual traffic conditions on roads. Hence, Google Maps may provide a more realistic

---

[1] https://developers.google.com/maps/documentation/staticmaps/. Last accessed on April 11, 2019.

driving time than a GIS. As there may be several routes between a city or town and a hospital in Google Maps, we tabulate the driving time for each selected city or town to all of the hospitals providing cardiac surgery services and select the route with the shortest driving time to approximate the service accessibility for the LHINs. *Service accessibility* is calculated by:

$$SA_i = \frac{\sum_{k=1}^{K_i} PS_{ki} * \psi_{ki}}{PS_i},$$ (3.3)

where SA_i is the service accessibility of LHIN i; PS_{ki} is the population size of a city/town k in LHIN i; K_i is the number of cities/towns selected in LHIN i; PS_i is the population size of LHIN i; and ψ_{ki} is a parameter denoting whether a city/town k in LHIN i is within a 30-min driving time to the nearest hospital. If the driving time from a city/town k in LHIN i to its nearest hospital is within 30 min, $\psi_{ki} = 1$; otherwise, $\psi_{ki} = 0$.

The geodemographic profiles of LHINs are summarized in Table 3.1.

The data representing cardiac surgery *service utilization* from 2004 to 2007 is obtained from the CCN.[2] Based on the CCN data, the average number of cardiac surgery patient arrivals in a hospital i each month over a quarter t (i.e., $A_i(t)$) can be calculated by adding the number of completed cases to the number of patients waiting in the queue (i.e., $Q_i(t)$), and subtracting the waiting queue length at time $t - 1$ (i.e., $Q(t - 1)$). An overview of the aggregated data on *service utilization* for each hospital is shown in Table 3.2.

Table 3.1 The measurement values for the geodemographic profiles of LHINs that have cardiac surgery services

LHIN ID	LHIN name	PS_i'	Age_i' (%)	SA_i (%)	E_i' (%)
2	South West	762,804	32.55	41.05	62.68
3	Waterloo Wellington	671,709	29.73	77.69	64.16
4	Hamilton Niagara Haldimand Brant	796,559	33.83	51.54	61.25
6	Mississauga Halton	912,292	27.54	88.20	71.51
7	Toronto Central	3,813,418	29.97	100.00	70.12
8	Central	637,510	30.07	75.13	69.35
10	South East	198,366	33.90	65.10	66.37
11	Champlain	651,966	32.80	86.40	74.16
13	North East	189,353	37.32	37.27	61.37

PS_i': the measurement value for *population size* of LHIN i, Age_i': the measurement value for *age profile* of LHIN i, SA_i: the measurement value for *service accessibility* of LHIN i, E_i': the measurement value for *educational profile* of LHIN i

[2]http://www.ccn.on.ca/ccn_public/FormsHome/HomePage.aspx. Last accessed on April 11, 2019.

Table 3.2 Cardiac surgery service utilization from 2004 to 2007 in Ontario hospitals

LHIN ID	Hospital	*Service utilization* (Mean)
2	London Health Sciences Centre	111
3	St. Mary's General Hospital	51
4	Hamilton Health Sciences	112
6	Trillium Health Partners	86
7	St. Michael's Hospital	88
7	Sunnybrook Health Sciences Centre	71
7	University Health Network	143
8	Southlake Regional Health Centre	64
10	Kingston General Hospital	53
11	University of Ottawa Heart Institute	91
13	Hôpital Régional de Sudbury Regional Hospital	38

3.3.2   Two-Step SEM Tests

The partial least squares (PLS)-based SEM software SmartPLS[3] is used to test the hypothesized relationships. PLS-based SEM, when compared with LISREL, another major type of SEM, has the advantage of theory development and thus is more appropriate for exploratory modeling [61]. In this study, all of the latent variables (LVs) (*population size, age profile, service accessibility, educational profile*, and *service utilization*) are modeled as reflective constructs, which are constructs viewed as causing, as opposed to being caused by, the observed variables [143].

We conduct a two-step test to test both the hypothesized direct and moderating effects.

- Step 1: Test the direct effects of *population size* and *age profile* on healthcare *service utilization*;
- Step 2: Explore the direct and the moderating effects of *educational profile* and *service accessibility* on *service utilization*.

3.3.3   Test Results

The research hypotheses are tested using secondary data on the service utilization of cardiac surgery in Ontario and the relevant geodemographic factors between 2004 and 2007 (16 quarters). The mean and standard deviation of the variables are summarized in Table 3.3.

---

[3]http://www.smartpls.de/. Last accessed on April 11, 2019.

Table 3.3 Summary statistics for the geodemographic factors and cardiac service utilization in Ontario between 2004 and 2007

Variable	Mean	Standard deviation	Min	Max
Population size	784,907	367,484	189,353	1,271,139
Age profile				
50+ (%)	31.60	2.63	27.54	37.32
Service accessibility				
≤30' (%)	67.90	19.59	37.27	100.00
Educational profile				
>High school (%)	67.38	4.24	61.25	74.16
Service utilization				
No. patient arrivals in a month	82	34	16	211

3.3.3.1 Measurement Model

The common evaluation metrics for model fitting in PLS-based SEM are Cronbach's alpha, construct reliability, and average variance extracted. As we use one observed variable for each LV, both Cronbach's alpha and the construct reliability of each LV are equal to 1, suggesting that all of the LVs are internally consistent [48]. The average variance extracted for each LV is also equal to 1, indicating adequate convergent validity [48]. Moreover, the correlations between each LV and the other LVs are smaller than the square root of the average variance extracted, indicating adequate discriminant validity [144].

3.3.3.2 The Effects of *Population Size* and *Age Profile* on *Service Utilization*

As Fig. 3.3 reveals, in support of **H1** and **H2**, both *population size* and *age profile* have significant positive effects on *service utilization*, with path coefficients of $\beta = 0.737$ (t = 13.205, $p < 0.01$) and $\beta = 0.284$ (t = 5.051, $p < 0.01$), respectively. These results support the previous findings that a larger population size [43, 65] and a greater proportion of residents older than 50 [133, 134] in a geographic area imply more cardiac surgery patients in the hospital(s) of that area.

3.3.3.3 The Effects of *Service Accessibility* and *Educational Profile* on *Service Utilization*

As Fig. 3.4 shows, in support of **H3.1** and **H3.2**, *service accessibility* is negatively related to *service utilization* ($\beta = -0.210$, t = 2.101, $p < 0.01$), and weakens the effect of *population size* on *service utilization* ($\beta = -0.606$, t = 5.240, $p < 0.01$). The findings suggest that the more accessible an LHIN is in terms of healthcare services (i.e., the more individuals within a 30-min driving time to the nearest hospital providing cardiac surgery services), the fewer the patient arrivals at any

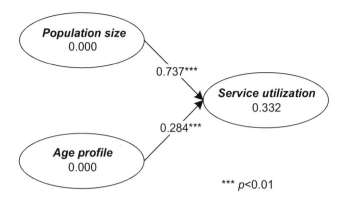

Fig. 3.3 SEM test results: the effects of *population size* and *age profile* on *service utilization*

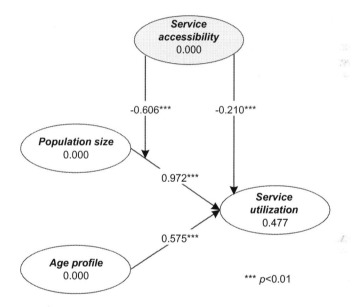

Fig. 3.4 SEM test results: *service accessibility* as a moderator

one hospital in this LHIN and the weaker the effect of *population size* on *service utilization*. However, **H3.3** is not supported by our data ($\beta = -0.070$, $t = 0.661$, $p > 0.05$), indicating that *service accessibility* does not have a moderating effect on the relationship between *age profile* and *service utilization*.

H4.1 is not supported by our data ($\beta = 0.050$, $t = 1.088$, $p > 0.1$), as shown in Fig. 3.5, suggesting that *educational profile* does not have a direct effect on patient *service utilization* for cardiac surgery. However, in support of **H4.2** and **H4.3**, our results reveal that *educational profile* weakens the effects of *population size* and *age profile* on *service utilization*, with path coefficients of $\beta = -0.595$ ($t = 7.592$,

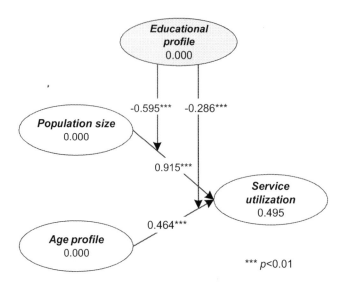

Fig. 3.5 SEM test results: *educational profile* as a moderator

Table 3.4 Hypothesis testing results

Hypotheses	Supported?
H1, H2, H3.1, H3.2, H4.2, H4.3	Fully supported
H3.3, H4.1	Not supported

$p < 0.01$) and $\beta = -0.286$ (t = 4.987, $p < 0.01$), respectively. The effects of *population size* and *age profile* on *service utilization* in a well-educated LHIN is therefore probably not as strong as in a less well-educated LHIN.

Table 3.4 summarizes the testing results for each of the hypotheses.

3.4 Discussion

Meeting the needs of a population is one of the most important considerations when allocating healthcare resources in Canada, and worldwide [130]. Previous research has advocated the allocation of resources according to the needs of the population, as assessed by an estimation method [130] that considers demographic-based indicators (e.g., age, education, and smoking) [145, 146]. However, Kephart and Asada [146] noted substantial differences between estimated and real service needs in some regions when examining traditional estimation methods. The needs estimation method may simply be a linear combination of all of the considered factors that does not consider how these factors interact with one another, resulting in a biased estimation. Therefore, an in-depth understanding of the direct and moderating interactions between the geodemographic factors and healthcare service utilization may suggest better estimation methods for healthcare service needs. LHINs are sub-provincial administrative units responsible for planning and funding healthcare services for their corresponding geographic areas in Ontario. By uncovering interesting relationships between LHINs' geodemographic factors and healthcare service utilization, we provide LHIN administrators with valuable information to consider in their planning and/or managing of healthcare service resources.

In the work presented in this study, we demonstrated that *service accessibility* has a significant moderating effect on the *population size-service utilization* relationship, and that *educational profile* exerts significant moderating effects on both the *population size-service utilization* relationship and the *age profile-service utilization* relationship. These relationships have not been reported previously. The results of our analysis confirm our prediction that *service accessibility* is negatively associated with *service utilization*, and that it weakens the effect of *population size* on *service utilization*. The results suggest that the more healthcare services are accessible in an area, the fewer cardiac surgery patient arrivals any one hospital in that area will have. We consider the Hamilton Niagara Haldimand Brant LHIN (LHIN 4) and its neighbor, the Mississauga Halton LHIN (LHIN 6), as examples. In 2007, the proportion of patients receiving cardiac surgery services in their resident LHINs (referred to as the inside-LHIN proportion) was 82% in LHIN 4 and 72% in LHIN 6 [136], whereas the service accessibility was approximately 51.54% in LHIN 4 and 88.20% in LHIN 6, as shown in Table 3.1. As both LHIN 4 and LHIN 6 have only one hospital in their own areas, the higher accessibility of LHIN 6 compared to LHIN 4 suggests that there are more accessible hospitals in the LHINs surrounding LHIN 6 than in those surrounding LHIN 4. As a result, patients dwelling in LHIN 4 are less likely to visit hospitals in other LHINs, compared to those dwelling in LHIN 6, and thus the inside-LHIN proportion for LHIN 4 is higher than that for LHIN 6. Accordingly, we expect that for LHINs with better accessibility to cardiac surgery services (e.g., LHINs 3, 6, 7, and 11, as shown in Table 3.1), the pressure of population growth in each of these LHINs on the hospital(s) within the LHIN may decrease.

In contrast, the negative but insignificant moderating effect of *service accessibility* on the relationship between the *age profile* and *service utilization* may be because older people are more willing to visit a familiar hospital or a hospital with familiar physicians [28]. Consequently, service accessibility in an LHIN, which reflects patients' options in healthcare services, may have little effect on the senior population's decisions when choosing cardiac surgery services.

The negative moderating effects of *educational profile* suggest that the effect of *population size* and *age profile* on *service utilization* is less pronounced in a well-educated population than it is in a less-educated population. Well-educated individuals, including the elderly, may have healthier lifestyles [14] and are more inclined to receive routine physical examinations and engage in self-care behavior [131]. Consequently, they are less likely to develop severe cardiovascular disease that requires cardiac surgery services [19]. As illustrated in Table 3.3, the educational profiles of the LHINs in 2006 vary from 61.25% to 74.16%, with a mean value of 67.38% and a standard deviation of 4.24%. The effects of population growth and aging on patient arrivals in each LHIN may therefore vary depending on the educational profiles of that LHIN. As shown in Table 3.1, LHINs 6, 7, 8, and 11, which have more educated populations (indicated by higher-than-average educational profiles), may have lower patient arrivals due to population growth and aging, compared to other LHINs.

Previous research has identified population growth and aging as two important factors driving the need for healthcare services in Ontario [18], and thus affecting patient arrivals. Likewise, our findings reveal a significant relationship between *population size* and *service utilization*, and between *age profile* and *service utilization*. This finding suggests that, monitoring the trends in population growth and aging is an effective precautionary approach for healthcare administrators aiming to provide sustainable healthcare services.

The literature has noted the significant positive effect that *service utilization* exerts on the important performance indicator of hospital wait times [42, 44]. Our findings suggest that geodemographic factors, such as *population size*, *age profile*, *service accessibility*, and *educational profile*, may indirectly affect wait times for cardiac surgery services via their influence on patient arrivals. Therefore, healthcare administrators should consider the roles of the geodemographic factors in their efforts to improve wait times for healthcare services.

In this chapter, we concentrate on four specific geodemographic factors, i.e., *population size*, *age profile*, *service accessibility*, and *educational profile*. These factors are identified based on a literature review and are not significantly correlated as tested on our aggregated data. It should be noted that there may be other geodemographic factors influencing *service utilization*, such as income, one of the commonly considered geodemographic characteristics in the literature. In this work, we do not pay attention to those factors because (1) some of them may significantly correlate with the *population size*, *age profile*, *service accessibility*, or *educational profile* (e.g., education attainment and income in a population have a causal relationship, as indicated by a few studies [147]); (2) the SEM test results show that approximately 50% of the variability in service utilization can be explained, suggesting that only considering the four factors in the data test is acceptable for they account for the major part of the variance in service utilization.

3.5 Summary

In this chapter, we demonstrated how to use the SEM-based analysis to explore the moderating effects of certain geodemographic factors, in addition to their direct effects, on healthcare service utilization. Unlike previous research, we used an SEM technique and aggregated data on geodemographic factors and cardiac surgery services in Ontario, Canada to test the hypothesized relationships. The results reveal that geodemographic changes due to population growth and aging may significantly affect cardiac surgery service utilization. Geographic accessibility to healthcare services and a population's educational profile exert significant effects on patient arrivals for cardiac surgery services, both as direct antecedents and as moderators. Our findings suggest the importance of considering the geodemographic profiles of a geographic area, and sometimes its neighboring areas, when allocating healthcare service resources, to strategically improve service utilization and reduce wait times. In addition, the work presented in this chapter demonstrates that the SEM-based analysis can be used to empirically identify the complex relationships between demand factors and wait times.

Chapter 4
Effects of Supply Factors on Wait Times

Prior research shows that supply factors, such as supplier capacity, significantly affect the throughput and the wait times within an isolated unit. However, it is doubtful whether the characteristics (i.e., service utilization, capacity, throughput, and wait times) of one unit affect the wait times of subsequent units on the patient flow process. To answer this question, this chapter examines the impact of characteristics of a catheterization unit (CU) on the wait times of a cardiac surgery unit (SU), within the scenario of cardiac care in Ontario, Canada. Figure 4.1a presents the research focus of this chapter within the overall framework of understanding a healthcare service system.

The work presented in this chapter gives an additional example of using *Structural Equation Modeling (SEM)-based analysis* to explore whether and how some supply factors affect wait times in a hospital. Following the steps of SEM-based analysis shown in Fig. 4.1b, we first propose research hypotheses and a corresponding conceptual model based on a literature review. We then test the hypotheses using SEM based on aggregated data that represents the characteristics of CUs and SUs in 11 hospitals in Ontario from 2005 to 2008. We finally discuss the interpretation of and possible extensions to our findings.

4.1 Introduction

The effect of highly fluctuating *service utilization* (represented by the number of patient arrivals, also called as *demand*) and available service *capacity* on the *performance* of a healthcare service system deserves long-standing attention [148, 149]. *Service utilization, capacity,* and *performance* are all important characteristics describing a healthcare service system. *Service utilization* is often represented by the number of visits to services [150, 151] or the expenditure on services [152, 153]. Some of the factors affecting the service utilization of a healthcare service system

© Springer Nature Switzerland AG 2019
L. Tao, J. Liu, *Healthcare Service Management*, Health Information Science,
https://doi.org/10.1007/978-3-030-15385-4_4

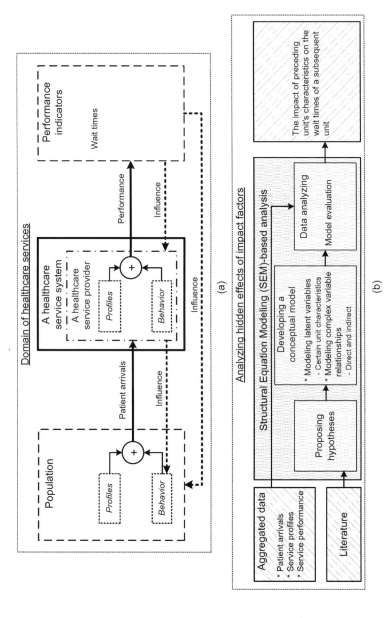

Fig. 4.1 A schematic diagram illustrating the use of an SEM-based analysis to examine the effect of a preceding unit's characteristics on the wait times of a subsequent unit. (**a**) The research focus of this chapter (highlighted in red) with respect to the larger context of understanding a healthcare service system. (**b**) Research steps of SEM-based analysis in this chapter

are increasing numbers of patients due to aging and a growing population [65], the incidence of specific diseases such as diabetes [154], the development of diagnostic and treatment technology [65], the position of the patient on a waiting list [155], the geographic distance between the patient and the services [21], patients' personal profiles (e.g., demographics [156] and socioeconomic condition [15, 157]), and unpredictable patient behavior like balking, reneging, jockeying, and repeating [96, 97, 158].

The *capacity* of a healthcare service system denotes the resources (e.g., financial, human, and physical) available to serve patients [159]. *Capacity* is usually judged by the quantity and quality of the resources at hand [29, 65] or the working time available [160]. Capacity is affected by factors such as human resources, for example skilled doctors and assistants (e.g., nurses, anesthetists) [29]; physical resources, for example beds and equipment [65]; management strategies, for example resource utilization and allocation [100]; and resource planning and scheduling [97, 100].

Performance is commonly summarized using *throughput* and *wait times* [20, 97, 161]. *Throughput* is typically quantified by counting the number of patients who have received a needed healthcare service in a given period [162]. It is thus a way to observe the use of healthcare service resources. Unlike *throughput, wait times* represent the amount of time patients have to wait before receiving needed healthcare services [20, 163]. Wait times are a particular concern in healthcare, especially for key services such as catheterization and cardiac surgery. A long wait is not only an impediment to quality care but also a risk factor for patients [164, 165]. There are various measurements for wait times, such as median wait times (i.e., the point at which half of the patients have received their treatment and the other half are still waiting) and queue length (i.e., the total number of patients in the waiting list) [20, 163]. *Wait times* differ depending on patient urgency categories. In a government dominated healthcare service system (e.g., Canada), each patient on the key units' waiting lists is assigned an urgency rating score according to the presenting symptoms [166, 167]. Wait times strategies are adopted based on different urgency categories [20]. The higher the urgent score patients have, the shorter time they will wait.

Prior research has empirically investigated the relationships between *service utilization, capacity, throughput,* and *wait times. Service utilization* has been shown to have a significant effect on *capacity* [168], *throughput,* and *wait times* in different units (e.g., a congested recovery room and an emergency department) [29, 42, 71]. *Capacity* has been found to have a positive effect on *service utilization,* that is, a higher capacity attracts more patients to a hospital, especially non-urgent patients [35, 39]. *Capacity* has also been discovered to exert a significant negative effect on *wait times* [29, 71, 169]. Although previous studies have suggested that improvements in throughput often accompany a reduction in wait times [170], the effect of *throughput* on *wait times* has not been empirically investigated.

Healthcare units and services have generally evolved in silos focusing on satisfying their own customers [171]. Accordingly, previous research has focused on the relationships between the characteristics within a specific unit. However, we argue that it is inadequate to examine the within-unit relationships in isolation

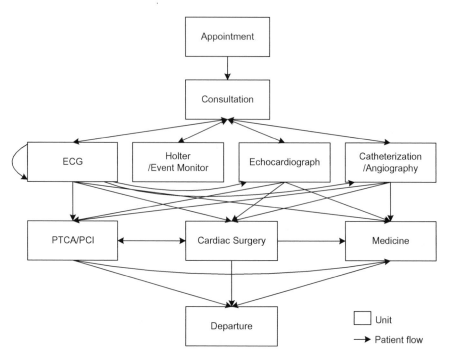

Fig. 4.2 The unit framework for cardiac care. ECG: Electrocardiogram; PTCA: Percutaneous Transluminal Coronary Angioplasty; PCI: Percutaneous Coronary Intervention

[171, 172], because, in the real world, all the units in a healthcare service system are networked via patient flow. For example, based on the cardiac treatment guideline [173], units involved in cardiac care are sequentially connected according to patient visits (as shown in Fig. 4.2). A directed link between two units denotes that they are temporally related, i.e., patients usually visit the unit the arrow points toward (i.e., the subsequent unit) after visiting the unit the arrow points away from (i.e., the preceding unit). There is usually a "funnel and filter effect" between two temporally related units, as preceding units "determine the absolute numbers of and speed of throughput for patients proceeding" into the subsequent units [174, p. 163]. In the context of cardiac care, a "diagnostic-therapeutic" cascade effect may also exist between a CU and a SU, as if more catheterization diagnostic tests are performed, more cardiac surgeries are likely to occur [175–177]. Thus, investigating the effect of cross-unit relationships, in addition to within-unit relationships, may reveal important insights for wait times management [172].

In summary, the impact factors for a unit's service performance, *wait times* and *throughput*, have been studied from the demand and the supply perspectives (as shown in Fig. 4.3). The relationships between *service utilization*, *capacity*, *throughput*, and *wait times* have been investigated within a unit. However, little attention has been paid to the relationships between the characteristics in a cross-unit context, a gap this study aims to fill. We use an SEM-based analysis to explore whether and how the characteristics of one unit exert an influence on the

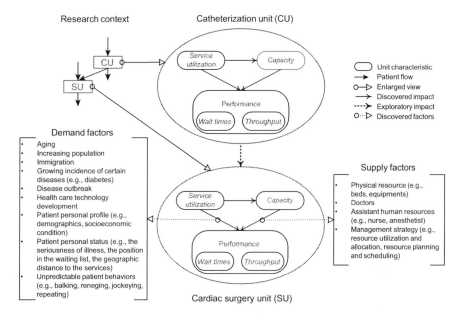

Fig. 4.3 The research framework summarizing the impact factors for throughput and wait times

characteristics of other temporally related units, focusing on *wait times* in particular. Figure 4.3 shows the overall research framework. We choose the CU and the SU as our research context because they both provide key services [20, 163]; they are temporally connected [178]; and published data on the two units are available.

4.2 The Effects of a Unit's Characteristics on Wait Times in a Subsequent Unit

Matching fluctuating patient arrivals for healthcare service systems with available capacity is known to be important for improving outcomes such as morbidity and mortality rate, as well as wait times [179]. Thus, there has been extensive research examining the relationships between *service utilization*, *capacity*, *throughput*, and *wait times*, especially within a single unit.

4.2.1 Hypotheses

4.2.1.1 Within-Unit Relationships

Prior research has shown that *service utilization* has a positive effect on *throughput* and *wait times*. For example, Asaro et al. [71] found that increasing patient arrivals in an emergency department (i.e., service utilization) also increased the throughput and wait times in the department. Schoenmeyr et al. [42] revealed a sensitive relationship between the caseload (i.e., service utilization) and the wait times in a congested recovery room. Harewood et al. [72] found that annual wait times for routine endoscopic procedures lengthened dramatically because of a significant increase in the demand for annual procedures on the endoscopy services. Therefore, we hypothesize that:

Hypothesis 1 (H1) *Service utilization* has a direct positive effect on *throughput* within a unit.

Hypothesis 2 (H2) *Service utilization* has a direct positive effect on *wait times* within a unit.

In analyzing the current research on the relationship between *service utilization* and *capacity*, Baker [168] noted that the desire to meet patient demands was a dominant driving force for capacity changing. Buerhaus [180] pointed out that service utilization increasing for aging population may result in an expanding nursing workforce (human resources) to avoid threatening the healthcare quality. Justman et al. [181] indicated that HIV scale-up is needed to develop laboratory systems and infrastructures (i.e., physical resources). Several researchers have argued that *capacity* has a positive effect on *service utilization* [35, 39]. For instance, Smethurst and Williams [39] noted that for each disease investigated, there were many more patients who did not visit the doctor than there were those who did visit (i.e., "latent" patients). To meet these potential overwhelming patient arrivals, the supplier may increase the system's capacity. Changes in the capacity may trigger changes in patient arrivals, because more patients are then attracted to that system. However, this argument has not been empirically tested [182]. We thus hypothesize that:

Hypothesis 3 (H3) *Service utilization* has a direct positive effect on *capacity* within a unit.

Prior research has indicated that *capacity* is important to ensure better performance in a healthcare service system, measured in *throughput* and *wait times*. For instance, Harindra et al. [29] found that supplier capacity was an important factor determining access inequalities (which is usually represented by wait times) in catheterization in Canada. Schoenmeyr et al. [42] showed that the physical capacity of a supplier (e.g., beds) had a significant effect on the wait times in a congested recovery room. Trzeciak and Rivers [169] also found that inpatient capacity (e.g., beds) had an effect on the throughput in an emergency department. Harewood et al. [72] further showed that modifications in routine clinical practice (i.e., service capacity) could significantly affect a procedure's wait times.

Some studies have revealed that improving *capacity* may help improve the *throughput* and the *wait times* in a unit. Mukherjee [183] found that improving the management of physicians (e.g., staffing mix) improved patient throughput. Others showed that improving capacity management (such as employing intelligent patient scheduling) shortened wait times efficiently [184, 185]. Therefore, we hypothesize that:

Hypothesis 4 (H4)   *Capacity* has a direct positive effect on *throughput* within a unit.

Hypothesis 5 (H5)   *Capacity* has a direct positive effect on *wait times* within a unit.

Few studies have investigated the relationship between *throughput* and *wait times*. Brenner et al. suggested that improvements in throughput are often accompanied by a reduction in wait times [170]. An intuitive explanation is that given stable patient arrivals (i.e., determined number of arrivals) in a unit, if resources (physical or human resources) in the unit can be more efficiently used, the patients may be treated quicker. So that the wait times of each patient may be shortened. Therefore, we hypothesize that:

Hypothesis 6 (H6)   *Throughput* has a direct negative effect on *wait times* within a unit.

4.2.1.2   Cross-Unit Relationships

Prior research has examined the relationships of characteristics among several units within a hospital. Alter et al. [174] reported that catheterization has a "funnel and filter" effect on cardiac surgery. Patient arrivals and the capacity of the CU therefore determine the absolute number of and speed of throughput for patients proceeding into the SU. Similarly, prior research has revealed that the CU and the SU have a "diagnostic and therapeutic" cascade effect [175–177]: if more catheterization diagnostic tests are performed in the CU, more patients may undergo cardiac surgeries. However, these studies do not explain clearly how and to what extent the capacity of one unit may influence the wait times of another. To the best of our knowledge, no prior study has examined whether and to what extent the wait times of one unit influences the wait times of a temporally related unit. We hypothesize that:

Hypothesis 7 (H7)   *Service utilization* of the CU has a positive effect on *service utilization* of the SU.

Hypothesis 8 (H8)   *Capacity* of the CU has a positive effect on *service utilization* of the SU.

Hypothesis 9 (H9)   *Wait times* in the CU have a positive effect on the *wait times* in the SU.

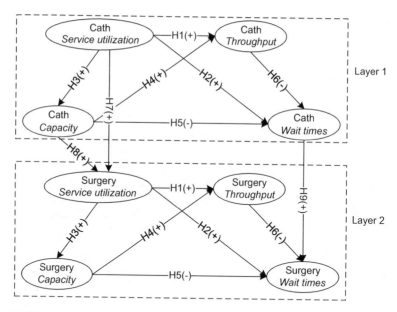

Fig. 4.4 The conceptual model for this study. Cath: catheterization; Surgery: cardiac surgery; H1–H9: research hypotheses; +/–: a positive or a negative relationship between two variables

4.2.2   The Conceptual Model

We postulate a conceptual two-layer wait times model, representing the hypothesized within-unit and cross-unit wait times relationships, as shown in Fig. 4.4. The relationships between four characteristics within the CU and the SU are illustrated in Layer 1 and Layer 2. Cross-unit wait times relationships are represented by the effects between the two layers.

4.3   SEM Tests and Results

4.3.1   Aggregated Data

The aggregated data used in this study was obtained from Cardiac Care Network (CCN), Ontario Physician Human Resources Data Center (OPHRDC), and College of Physicians and Surgeons of Ontario (CPSO) in Ontario, Canada. The reported data from CCN includes the number of completed cases in a month, the average number of patients waiting at the end of a month, and the monthly average median wait times for each hospital. We are particularly interested in the units of catheterization and cardiac surgery, because a regional priority rating score system has been established for these two units (but not other units) in Ontario [166, 167]. The CCN thus provides more detailed statistics for the CU and SU than for other

Table 4.1 Cardiac surgery statistics from January 2008 to March 2008 in Ontario hospitals

Hospital	C	UM (d)	SM (d)	EM (d)	Q
London Health Sciences Centre	115	2	5	17	33
St. Mary's General Hospital	61	3	5	9	24
Hamilton Health Sciences	127	1	6	12	69
Trillium Health Partners	79	2	4	9	22
St. Michael's Hospital	89	5	6	15	26
Sunnybrook HSC	56	3	4	16	22
University Health Network	129	2	6	13	135
Southlake Regional HC	75	5	7	28	42
Kingston General Hospital	47	3	15	20	30
University of Ottawa Heart Institute	98	6	21	52	100
Hôpital Régional de Sudbury Regional Hospital	36	7	6	19	21

C: the number of completed cases; UM: median wait times for urgent patients; SM: median wait times for semi-urgent patients; EM: median wait times for elective patients; Q: the number of patients waiting at the end of a month; d: days

units. Table 4.1 shows the major information provided in the CCN report. From Table 4.1, we can observe the variability of the throughput and the wait times for a specific unit.

We propose an equation as follows to calculate the monthly average number of arrivals from the existing statistic data, so that the demands of CU and SU can be estimated successfully.

$$A_i(t) = B_i(t) + Q_i(t) - Q_i(t - 1), \tag{4.1}$$

where, $A_i(t)$ is the monthly average number of arrivals in quarter t in unit i, $B_i(t)$ is the monthly average number of patients who have received treatment in quarter t in unit i, and $Q_i(t)$ is the average number of patients waiting at the end of a month in quarter t in unit i.

The capacity of SUs is precisely measured by the number of physicians who specialize in cardiac surgery. The capacity of CUs is approximately measured by the number of physicians who perform diagnostic radiology, because catheterization is one of the tests that uses radiology, and information about the physicians who perform catheterization is unavailable. However, since the OPHRDC data is organized by LHINs, not by hospitals, it needs to be processed so as to align with the CCN data. Table 1.2 shows the CCN member hospitals and the corresponding LHINs. From this table, we can see direct correspondences between the LHINs and CCN member hospitals, except the LHINs of Toronto Central (TC) and North East (NE), which have more than one CCN hospital. To facilitate data analysis, the two LHINs' data should be decomposed to generate data for related hospitals.

The main idea behind data decomposition is to utilize hospitals' physician ratio (calculated from the number of specific physicians in a hospital to the total number of the specific physicians in the corresponding LHIN in year of 2010) in TC and

Table 4.2 A summary of the characteristics of the CU and SU

Characteristics	Measurements	CU	SU
Service utilization	Monthly number of arrivals	340	82
Capacity	Number of physicians, yearly	60	7
Throughput	Monthly number of completed patients	346	83
Wait times	Median wait times of U/S/E patients	1/10/15	3/6/19
	Number of waits at the end of a month	101	58

CU: Catheterization unit; *SU*: Cardiac surgery unit; *U*: urgent; *S*: semi-urgent; *E*: elective

NE to compute the number of physicians for relevant hospitals from 2005 to 2008. The physician ratios for CU and SU in each hospital in TC and NE can be obtained from CPSO. Then, after observing the OPHRDC data, we found that in TC and NE, the changes in CU ranged from 0 to 9 physicians per LHIN year to year (the total average number of catheterization physicians per hospital in the two LHINs was 60); and the changes in SU ranged from 0 to 1 physician per LHIN year to year (the total average number of cardiac surgery physicians per hospital in the two LHINs was 7). Therefore, we can assume that the physician ratios in TC and NE are relatively stable, i.e., the physician ratios are the same in each year since 2005. So that the number of specific physicians in each hospital can be calculated successfully by the specific physician ratio of each hospital multiplied by the number of the specific physicians in the corresponding LHIN each year.

By integrating and processing the two sets of data as discussed above, we obtain comprehensive information about the 11 hospitals (enumerated in Table 4.1) that provide catheterization and cardiac surgery. Table 4.2 outlines the characteristics of the two units and their measurements with the data summary. Specifically, we focus on the data from 2005 to 2008 (15 quarters in total), because the year of 2004 is the end of the first 6-year cardiac expansion plan [65] and the start of the second 10-year cardiac improvement plan [20, 186]. In total, there are 165 data points for CU and SU (one hospital one quarter is regarded as a data point). In the next subsection, we will describe the statistical analysis methods used to investigate within-unit and cross-unit wait times relationships.

4.3.2 SEM Tests

We use PLS-based SEM [61] to test the proposed two-layer wait times model (shown in Fig. 4.4) and the related hypotheses as this study is exploratory rather than confirmatory. The software SmartPLS[1] is used for path modeling and PLS-based data analysis.

In SEM-based data analysis, the measurements for *wait times* are modeled as formative indicators rather than reflective ones [61, 143]. A formative model is used when a latent construct (i.e., a factor, such as *service utilization*, *capacity*,

---

[1]http://www.smartpls.de/. Last accessed on April 11, 2019.

throughput, and *wait times*) is viewed as an explanatory combination of its manifest variables (i.e., measurements) [144, 187]. In contrast, in a reflective model, the manifest variables are viewed as being caused by a underlying common dimension or a construct [187]. Here, the manifest variables for *wait times* are not interchangeable or correlated with one another because they measure *wait times* from different perspectives. Therefore, the LV *wait times* is the summation of its corresponding manifest variables. In other words, the measurement items of *wait times* will be formative in the construct of *wait times*.

We use the data for the CU and SU in the same quarter to test the cross-unit relationships. As the longest waiting time for a patient in the CU is around one month, we can assume that the great majority of patients who need cardiac surgery will be transferred from the CU to the SU within a quarter. In the next section, we present the results of the PLS analysis, focusing on how the characteristics affect one another within a unit and how the characteristics of the CU affect the characteristics of the SU, particularly the SU's *wait times*.

4.3.3 Test Results

4.3.3.1 Within-Unit Relationships

As illustrated in Fig. 4.5, in support of H1–H3, *service utilization* has a significant positive effect on *throughput*, *capacity*, and *wait times*. The path coefficients for the effect of *service utilization* on *throughput* are $\beta = 0.585$ (t $= 18.677$, $p < 0.01$) for the CU and $\beta = 0.797$ ($t = 35.115$, $p < 0.01$) for the SU. The path coefficients for the effect of *service utilization* on *capacity* are $\beta = 0.921$ (t $= 127.754$, $p < 0.01$) for the CU and $\beta = 0.574$ (t $= 25.219$, $p < 0.01$) for the SU. The path coefficients for the effect of *service utilization* on *wait times* are $\beta = 0.619$ (t $= 2.908$, $p < 0.05$) for the CU and $\beta = 0.472$ (t $= 6.111$, $p < 0.01$) for the SU. These results confirm findings from prior studies [29, 42, 71, 72, 168], providing further evidence that *service utilization* is an important predictor for *capacity*, *throughput* and *wait times* within a unit.

In support of H4, *capacity* has a significant positive effect on *throughput*. The path coefficients for the effect of *capacity* on *throughput* are $\beta = 0.410$ (t $= 13.162$, $p < 0.01$) for the CU and $\beta = 0.155$ (t $= 5.914$, $p < 0.01$) for the SU. These results also confirm findings from prior studies [169, 183], suggesting that an improvement in capacity will lead to improved throughput within a unit.

Hypothesis H5 is only partially supported by our data. For the CU, *capacity* has a significant negative effect on *wait times* ($\beta = -0.252$, t $= 2.465$, $p < 0.01$), thus supporting H5. However, for the SU, *capacity* has a significant positive effect on *wait times* ($\beta = 0.115$, t $= 3.071$, $p < 0.01$), which does not support H5. This finding differs with prior studies [42, 72], which suggests that an improvement in a unit's capacity can significantly shorten its patients' wait times.

The positive effect of *capacity* on *wait times* for the SU can be explained using Smethurst and Williams's work [35, 39]. They found that hospital waiting lists are

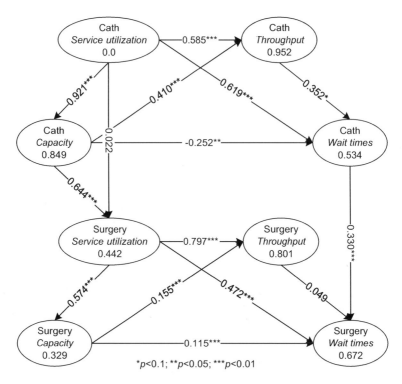

Fig. 4.5 PLS test results based on a formative measurement model. Cath: catheterization; Surgery: cardiac surgery

self-regulating. When capacity increases to meet the needs of patients, the number of patient arrivals may change again, creating an even greater number of patient arrivals. A mass of "hidden" patients [39] who have diseases but have not been willing to go to a hospital, may be persuaded to visit that hospital if they believe that they will be treated quicker. Hence, expanding the capacity of the SU may help shorten wait times temporarily, but the wait times will then increase beyond their initial values, as patient arrivals increase in response to the larger capacity.

Hypothesis H6 is not supported by our data. *Throughput* has a significant positive effect on *wait times* ($\beta = 0.352$, t $= 1.659$, $p < 0.1$) in the CU, whereas the effect of *throughput* on *wait times* is negligible for the SU ($\beta = 0.049$, t $= 0.593$, $p > 0.1$). This finding suggests that *throughput* and *wait times* have similar changing patterns in the CU, but not in the SU, which is contrary to the expectation that an improvement in the throughput will result in an improvement in wait times.

Urgent patients' queue jumping behavior may explain the positive relationship between *throughput* and *wait times* in the CU. Queue jumping means that urgent patients can skip the queue and jump to any position on a waiting list because of their treatment priority [188]. If more urgent patients arrive, units delay the treatment of the semi-urgent and elective patients to serve the high priority patients in time, indirectly making the non-urgent patients wait longer. The overall wait times for the unit may increase as a result. The absence of a significant relationship between the *throughput* and *wait times* in the SU could be because the SU has much fewer urgent patients than the CU does. For instance, in the fiscal year of 2004, the percentage of urgent patients in the CU in Ontario was 49% (out of a total of 52,628 patients), whereas the percentage of urgent patients in the SU was only 23% (out of a total of 7825 patients) [20]. This finding implies that, in some cases, *throughput* and *wait times* may not be directly related to reflect the quality of a unit's performance.

4.3.3.2 Cross-Unit Relationships

As show in Fig. 4.5, H7 is not supported by our data ($\beta = 0.022$, t $= 0.277$, $p >$ 0.1). The *service utilization* of the CU does not have a significant effect on the *service utilization* of the SU. The *capacity* of the CU has a significant positive effect on the *service utilization* of the SU ($\beta = 0.644$, t $= 8.498$, $p < 0.01$), which supports H8.

These two findings explain the formation of the "funnel and filter" effect [174] between the CU and the SU. They suggest that more arrivals in the CU usually lengthen the waiting list, but do not heavily affect the throughput proceeding to the SU. In reality, the CU always has a waiting list, as can be seen in the CCN data. However, the capacity of the CU heavily determines the absolute number of and speed of throughput for patients proceeding into the SU, forming the "funnel and filter".

In support of H9, the results of our analysis reveal that the *wait times* in the CU have a significant positive effect on the *wait times* in the SU ($\beta = 0.330$, t $=$ 9.859, $p < 0.01$). This is strong evidence that the *wait times* in the CU are an important predictor for the *wait times* in the SU. A possible explanation for this effect is a delay cascade [189]. Unnikrishnan et al. [189] simulated and observed that delays will cascade in an emergency department network. In that study, all of the emergency departments in different hospitals were networked by the transfer paths of ambulances). In other words, delays in an emergency department will result in the wait times increasing in other emergency departments nearby. Cardiac care has a similar unit network (shown in Fig. 4.2) in a hospital. Therefore, delays in one unit may spread to other related units in the unit network, forming the direct cross-unit wait times relationship.

Table 4.3 summarizes the hypothesis testing results. An examination of our results, shown in Fig. 4.5, reveals both direct and indirect causal paths from the characteristics of the CU to the *wait times* in the SU. The *service utilization* and *capacity* of the CU also have indirect effect on the *wait times* in the SU, in addition to the direct effects. In other words, the *wait times* in the SU may be influenced by the CU via the following causal paths: *wait times* in the CU → *wait times* in the SU; *service utilization* of the CU → *capacity* of the CU → *service utilization* of the SU → *wait times* in the SU; and *service utilization* of the CU → *capacity* of the CU → *service utilization* of the SU → *capacity* of the SU → *wait times* in the SU. The *service utilization* of the CU appears to be the most essential driving force for the wait times dynamics in the CU and in the SU.

Table 4.3 Hypothesis testing results

Hypotheses	Supported?
H1–H4, H8, H9	Fully supported
H5	Partially supported
H6, H7	Not supported

4.4 Discussion

In this chapter, we have examined whether and how the characteristics of a preceding unit can affect the *wait times* in the SU. Unlike prior studies, we used SEM to assess the cross-unit wait times relationships from data published on healthcare services in Ontario, Canada. The results of our analysis validate the proposed conceptual model, thus providing empirical support for the hypothesized relationships between the characteristics *service utilization, capacity, throughput,* and *wait times,* both within a unit and across units.

Our results show that the *wait times* in the CU have a direct positive effect on the *wait times* in the SU. This is a novel result, as prior research has seldom examined the influence of one unit's *wait times* on the *wait times* in a subsequent unit in the patient flow process. A possible explanation for the effect is a delay cascade in the cardiac care unit network (Fig. 4.2), proposed by Unnikrishnan et al. [189].

The results of our analysis provide empirical evidence for previous findings that within a unit, *service utilization* has a positive effect on *capacity, throughput,* and *wait times;* within a unit, *capacity* has a positive effect on *throughput;* and that across units, the *service utilization* of one unit will be positively influenced by the *capacity* of the preceding unit.

We also obtained the surprising findings that the relationship between *capacity* and *wait times* differs in units with different profiles (e.g., different patient proportion in each urgency category); *throughput* has a positive effect on the *wait times* in a unit; there are direct and indirect wait times relationships between temporally-related units; and that *service utilization* of the CU is an essential predictor for the other characteristics of the CU and SU.

However, there may be other factors affecting a unit's performance in addition to *service utilization, capacity,* and cross-unit relationships. For example, the patient *risk* profile (i.e., the value of predicted operative mortality) has been identified as a factor that may affect triage or referral patterns and the allocation of resources [190]. Although the exact effects of patient risk profiles on service performance (*wait times* in particular) are still unclear, these relationships should be explored by incorporating patient risk into our conceptual model.

There are different methods for calculating the value of risk for patients undergoing catheterization (e.g., SYNTAX[2]) and cardiac surgery (e.g., EuroSCORE[3] and Higgins Score [191]) based on several risk factors. For example, the surgical risk

---

[2]http://www.syntaxscore.com/. Last accessed on April 11, 2019.

[3]http://www.euroscore.org/. Last accessed on April 11, 2019.

factors for isolated coronary artery bypass graft (CABG) surgery include age, sex, precious CABG, left ventricular function, and coronary anatomy, among others. [178, 192]. The Institute for Clinical Evaluative Science of Ontario has published data on the distribution of risk profiles in isolated CABG, the major type of cardiac surgery, in 2005 and 2006 in Ontario hospitals [178]. We used this published risk profile data (represented by the percentage of low-, medium-, and high-risk patients for catheterization in a hospital), to investigate the relationship between *risk* profiles and *wait times*. The missing data for each hospital's risk profiles for 2007 and 2008 are substituted with the mean value of the available risk data for that hospital [178], which is a common method for handling missing data in statistical data analysis [193, 194]. By integrating our original cardiac care data with the risk profile data, we conduct an additional PLS analysis to test the extended two-layer wait times model, with risk profiles added as an extra predictor of wait times in the SU (see Figs. 4.6, 4.7, and 4.8).

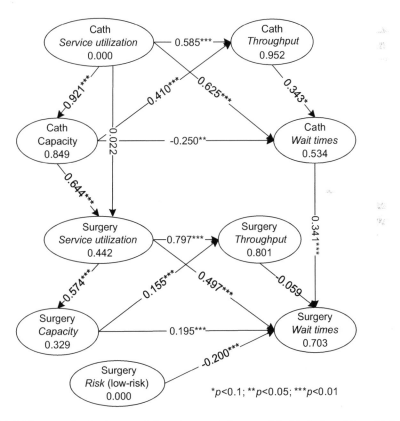

Fig. 4.6 PLS test results for the extended two-layer wait times model with the low-risk profile in the SU. Cath: catheterization; Surgery: cardiac surgery

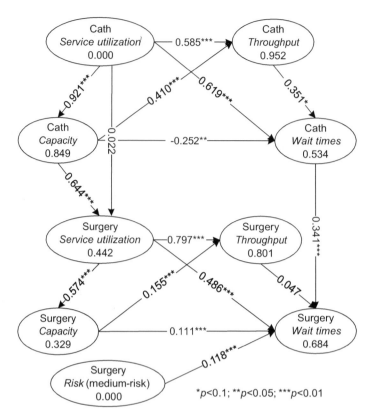

Fig. 4.7 PLS test results for the extended two-layer wait times model with the medium-risk profile in the SU. Cath: catheterization; Surgery: cardiac surgery

The results of the analysis (Figs. 4.6, 4.7, and 4.8) reveal that the pattern of within- and cross-unit relationships (i.e., hypotheses H1–H9) between characteristics (i.e., *service utilization*, *capacity*, *throughput*, and *wait times* in the CU and SU) remain unchanged. When *risk* profiles are represented differently, as a percentage of *low-risk* patients, percentage of *medium-risk* patients, or percentage of *high-risk* patients, they can have different effects on the *wait times* in the SU.

The percentage of *low-risk* patients has a significant negative effect on *wait times* (see Fig. 4.6). The explanation for this finding is still unclear as almost no prior work has addressed this issue to the best of our knowledge. However, we postulate that the treatment process for low-risk patients is easier than for higher-risk patients, and hence, the length of stay (including the pre-operative, operating, and post-operative stay) of low-risk patients may be shorter than higher-risk patients. Therefore, if there are more low-risk patients in the SU, the total wait times in this unit will decrease.

Interestingly, the percentage of *medium-risk* patients has a significant positive effect on *wait times* (see Fig. 4.7). This may be due to unexpected upgrading of the patients proceeding to cardiac surgery to more urgent categories (e.g., upgrading the

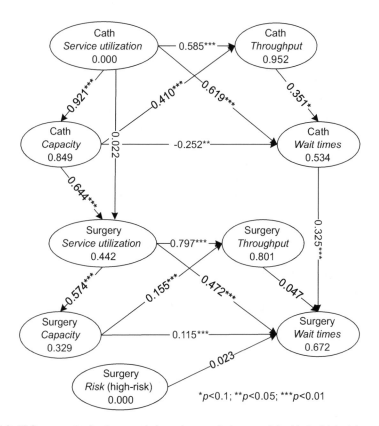

Fig. 4.8 PLS test results for the extended two-layer wait times model with the high-risk profile in the SU. Cath: catheterization; Surgery: cardiac surgery

medium-risk patients from semi-urgent to urgent) [195, 196]. The upgrading event may trigger queue jumping behavior [188], which will hinder the normal treatment schedule and result in longer wait times. This observation is consistent with the prior findings that proportionately more patients in the more urgent categories than in the less urgent categories may have wait times in excess of the maximum acceptable [197].

The percentage of *high-risk* patients does not have a significant effect on *wait times* (see Fig. 4.8), contrary to our expectation. Prior work indicates that high-risk patients tend to be assigned higher priorities in the triage process [195], and thus more high-risk patients may imply more urgent patients. As urgent patients are more likely to undergo expedited surgery, treatment for non-urgent patients may be delayed, resulting in prolonged overall wait times [188]. Although, we do not yet have a sound explanation for this unexpected lack of effect, the observed inconsistency between the effect of the high-risk profile and that of the medium-risk profile may be due to the methodology used to stratify the patient risk profiles and priority categories, an issue that deserves further investigation.

4.5   Summary

In this chapter, we demonstrated an additional example of using the method of SEM-based analysis to examine whether and how the characteristics of a preceding unit exerts an effect on the wait times in subsequent units. Focusing on cardiac care services, we investigated two temporally related units in cardiac care, the CU and its subsequent unit, the SU. Our results reveal that *wait times* in the CU has a direct positive effect on *wait times* in the SU; *capacity* of the CU has a direct positive effect on *service utilization* of the SU. Within each unit, there are significant relationships between the characteristics, except for the effect of *throughput* on *wait times* in the SU; different patient *risk* profiles may affect the *wait times* in the SU in different ways (e.g., positive or negative effects). The findings presented in this chapter suggest that when healthcare administrators seek to alleviate wait times in a healthcare service system, they should consider the cross-unit wait times relationships and take into account the relationship between priority triage and risk stratification, especially for cardiac surgery. The work presented in this chapter once again demonstrates that the SEM-based analysis is effective in identifying the complex relationships between multiple observed variables and LVs.

Chapter 5
Integrated Prediction of Service Performance

Estimating the changes of patient arrivals and service performance over the mid- or long-term is a common problem faced by healthcare service managers. To address this problem, we should know what factors result in the changes of the patient arrivals and service performance. How do these factors change in the future? How do the patient arrivals and service performance change in accordance with the variations of these factors? Figure 5.1a shows the research focus in this chapter with respect to the larger context of understanding a healthcare service system.

This chapter presents an example to show how to use our proposed *integrated prediction* method for predicting the changes of the healthcare service performance with respect to demographic shifts in the context of cardiac surgery services in Ontario, Canada. As illustrated in Fig. 5.1b, the *integrated prediction* method consists of the following three steps: (1) applying the *Structural Equation Modeling (SEM)-based analysis* to identify the complex relationships between demographic profiles and healthcare service characteristics (e.g., capacity, supply, utilization, and performance); (2) carrying out the *prediction* to estimate the service utilization and service performance based on the discovered complex relationships and demographic shifts; and (3) conducting the *queueing model analysis* to gain insights into the changing patterns of the estimated service performance over time. The work presented in this chapter shows that the proposed method gives a way to reasonably estimate the variations in service utilization and service performance with respect to the changes of certain factors.

5.1   Introduction

Many areas in the world now face notable demographic changes/shifts due to aging and immigration [129, 198]. For example, it was projected that the population aged 65 and above in Ontario, Canada, would increase from 1.8 million in 2010

© Springer Nature Switzerland AG 2019
L. Tao, J. Liu, *Healthcare Service Management*, Health Information Science,
https://doi.org/10.1007/978-3-030-15385-4_5

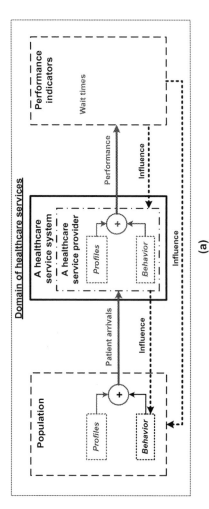

(a)

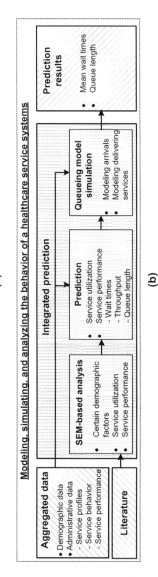

(b)

Fig. 5.1 A schematic diagram illustrating the use of integrated prediction to predict the changes in service performance with respect to demographic shifts. (**a**) The research focus of this chapter (highlighted in red) with respect to the larger context of understanding a healthcare service system. (**b**) Research steps of using an integrated prediction method to forecast service performance in this chapter

to 4.1 million in 2036, accounting for 13.9% and 23.4% of the total population, respectively [128]. The number of new immigrants in Ontario was predicted to increase by 0.107–0.135 million annually from 2010 to 2036, accounting for nearly 70% of the total population growth [128].

Demographic shifts (e.g., age and ethnic profiles) are known to have a direct effect on healthcare service utilization due to their correlations with risk factors for certain diseases and with service utilization behavior. For example, risk factors associated with cardiovascular diseases are more prevalent in the population aged 50 years old and above [13, 19]. Ethnic groups differ in their risks for cardiovascular diseases [19, 49, 199] and in their healthcare service utilization behavior [200, 201].

Demographic shifts will also have an effect on the performance (i.e., throughput and wait times) of a healthcare service. It has been found that healthcare service performance is affected not only by supply factors, such as physical and human resources, and management strategies [51, 202], but also by the dynamics of patient arrivals in terms of volume and characteristics (e.g., patient profile and severity of diseases with various co-morbidities) [44, 202]. An in-depth understanding of the potential changes in healthcare service characteristics (e.g., service utilization and performance) due to demographic changes will be helpful for middle-/long-term healthcare resource planning and allocation.

In view of this, in this chapter, we attempt to address the following research questions.

- The relationships between demographic profiles and healthcare service utilization involve several factors with direct and/or indirect, linear and/or nonlinear, and dynamic interactions. How can we learn these multi-factor complex relationships from limited aggregated data?
- Once we have found the multi-factor complex relationships between demographic profiles and healthcare service utilization, how can we predict the changes in service utilization with respect to demographic shifts?
- Estimation results based on multi-factor complex relationships are somewhat uncertain and cannot demonstrate the dynamics of estimated service utilization over time. How can we determine the dynamically changing process of healthcare service utilization with respect to demographic shifts?

To answer these questions, we propose a method of *integrated prediction*. This method uses an *SEM-based analysis* to discover the complex effects of multiple factors on service utilization and service performance, carries out a *prediction* to estimate healthcare service utilization based on the derived multi-factor complex relationships, and constructs a *queueing model* to simulate the dynamics of the estimated performance over time.

We apply the integrated prediction method to estimate the changes in service utilization and service performance in cardiac surgery services in Ontario, Canada. Our method is shown to be able to identify the complex relationships between the age profile, recent immigrant (RI) profile, and characteristics of cardiac surgery; describe the variations in healthcare service utilization with respect to demographic shifts; and demonstrate the temporal changes in estimated cardiac surgery performance using queueing model simulations.

5.2   Integrated Prediction

We propose an analytical method (shown in Fig. 5.2) to unveil the underlying relationships between demographic shifts and healthcare service utilization.

1. *Analysis of complex relationships between factors*: Based on a training data set (e.g., statistics), we use SEM [48] to identify the complex relationships between multiple factors (e.g., the age and recent immigrant profiles, and cardiac surgery characteristics in our case study).
2. *Qualitative prediction*: Based on the identified multi-factor complex relationships from the first step, we propose a set of equations to estimate the changes in service utilization with respect to demographic shifts.
3. *Dynamics simulation*: Based on the estimated service utilization, we build specific queueing models to simulate the operation of different healthcare services, such as cardiac surgery operating rooms (CS-ORs) in our case study, to gain insights into the performance dynamics of their provided services over time.

5.2.1   SEM-Based Analysis

SEM uses a measurement model and a structural model to explore the complex relationships between factors/variables (as shown in Fig. 5.3). The measurement model [48] characterizes the linear relationships between observed measurement variables (MVs) and the corresponding latent variables (LVs). One of the typical ways to relate MVs to LVs is through the reflective measurement model, in which each LV is reflected in its corresponding MV. Formally, let $\Xi = \{\xi_1, \xi_2, \ldots, \xi_N\}$ be a set of LVs and $X_{\xi_j} = \{x_{j1}, x_{j2}, \ldots, x_{N_\xi M_{\xi_j}}\}$ be a set of MVs relating to ξ_j ($\forall j \in [1, N_\xi]$), where $N_\xi = |\Xi|$ denotes the total number of LVs and $M_{\xi_j} = |X_{\xi_j}|$ denotes the total number of MVs which relate to ξ_j ($\forall j \in [1, N_\xi]$). The relationship between x_{jk} ($\forall k \in [1, M_{\xi_j}]$) and its related ξ_j can be expressed as follows [203]:

$$x_{jk} = \pi_{jk0} + \pi_{jk}\xi_j + \varepsilon_{jk}, \qquad (5.1)$$

where π_{jk0} and π_{jk} (i.e., loading in SEM) are the regression parameters and ε_{jk} is the residual error.

The structural model [48] describes the linear relationships between the LVs. Formally, let $\tilde{\Xi}_{\xi_j}$ ($\tilde{\Xi}_{\xi_j} \subset \Xi$) be a set of LVs that ξ_j relates to. The relationships

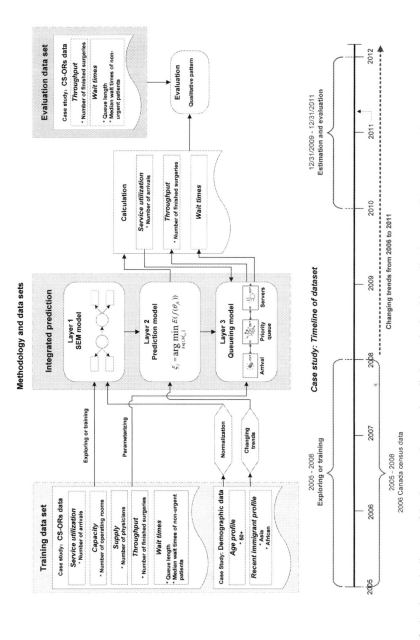

Fig. 5.2 A schematic diagram of the three-step integrated prediction method and its application to cardiac surgery services

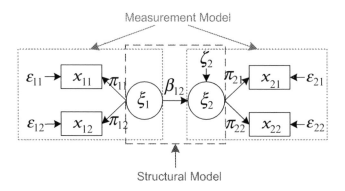

Fig. 5.3 The basic components in SEM

between ξ_j ($\xi_j \in \Xi$) and its related LVs ($\tilde{\Xi}_{\xi_j}$) can be written as follows [203]:

$$\xi_j = \beta_{j0} + \sum_i \beta_{ji}\xi_i + \zeta_j, \tag{5.2}$$

where β_{j0} is a constant number, β_{ji} (i.e., the path coefficient in SEM) is the regression weight of ξ_i ($\forall \xi_i \in \tilde{\Xi}_{\xi_j}$) relating to ξ_j, and ζ_j is the residual error.

We test multi-factor complex relationships using Partial Least Squares (PLS)-based SEM, as it is more suitable for exploratory studies, as in this study, than covariance-based SEM [61].

5.2.2 Prediction

In this subsection, we describe how to estimate healthcare service utilization based on demographic shifts and multi-factor complex relationships. The estimation process follows four sub-steps.

S1: Calculating the value of any exogenous LV with respect to the change in each corresponding MV using Eq. 5.3. An exogenous LV ξ_j ($\xi_j \in \Xi$) is an LV that does not vary due to other LVs.

$$\xi'_j = f(\theta_{jk}|\pi_{jk}, \sigma_{jk}, \Delta x_{jk}) = \frac{x_{jk}(1 + \Delta x_{jk})^\tau}{\pi_{jk}} - \sigma_{jk} + \theta_{jk}, \tag{5.3}$$

where ξ'_j is the estimation value of ξ_j given the changes in its MV; $\sigma_{jk} = \frac{\pi_{jk0} + \varepsilon_{jk}}{\pi_{jk}}$ represents a constant value; Δx_{jk} is the changing rate of x_{jk} per time unit; and θ_{jk} represents how ξ_j will change in accordance with a variation in x_{jk}.

S2: Taking an estimation value for each exogenous LV based on Eq. 5.4. Let X'_{ξ_j} $(X'_{\xi_j} \subseteq X_{\xi_j})$ be a set of changed MVs related to an exogenous LV ξ_j, and let $M'_{\xi_j} = |X'_{\xi_j}|$ denote the number of MVs that change in the estimation time τ. As each exogenous LV, ξ_j, has $|X'_{\xi_j}|$ estimated values in accordance with the changes in the MVs X'_{ξ_j}, we minimize the expectation of θ_{jk} ($k \in [1, M'_{\xi_j}]$) to get one reasonable estimation value for the exogenous LV, ξ_j.

$$\xi'_j = \arg \min_{k \in [1, M'_{\xi_j}]} E(f(\theta_{jk}|\pi_{jk}, \sigma_{jk}, \Delta x_{jk})). \tag{5.4}$$

It should be noted that if all of the MVs related to an exogenous LV, ξ_j, do not change during the estimation time τ, then the estimation value of ξ_j, i.e., ξ'_j, will be equal to the original value of ξ_j discovered by SEM.

S3: Calculating any endogenous LV, ξ_j ($\xi_j \in \Xi$), with Eq. 5.5, based on the multi-factor complex relationships learned by SEM. An endogenous LV is an LV which varies depending on other LVs.

$$\xi'_j = \beta_{j0} + \sum_i \beta_{ji} \xi'_i + \zeta_j, \tag{5.5}$$

where ξ'_j is the estimated value of ξ_j given the estimated values of its related LVs, $\tilde{\Xi}_{\xi_j}$.

S4: Calculating the MVs related to each endogenous LV using Eq. 5.1.

5.2.3 Queueing Model Simulation

Queueing models are useful for simulating the operation of healthcare systems and investigating interrelated processes, such as arriving at a queue and waiting [42, 54, 96]. A general queueing model (as shown in Fig. 5.4) for simulating a healthcare service system should define the following four basic characteristics.

- *Patient types and arrival patterns* (commonly denoted by λ): Patients to specific healthcare services can be divided into different types according to their characteristics. For example, as shown in Fig. 5.4, patients are usually categorized as urgent, semi-urgent, and elective. Different patient groups may differ in arrival rates and received services, such as service priority and service time. The arrival pattern is usually represented by a statistical distribution of inter-arrival times.
- *Patient behavior*: Some patients may be sensitive to wait times and may quit a queue if they have to wait too long, whereas others may be willing to stay in a queue no matter how long they will wait. This patient behavior may affect the performance of a healthcare service system and thus should be stated clearly in modeling.

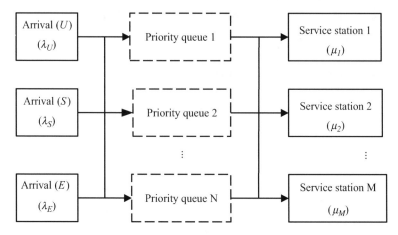

Fig. 5.4 A schematic diagram of a general queueing model for healthcare. E: elective, S: semi-urgent, U: urgent

- *Service capacity and service patterns* (commonly denoted by μ): In a healthcare service system, the service capacity usually corresponds to the number of service stations (e.g., the number of ORs). The service behavior usually exhibits specific patterns. For instance, the service time for patients normally follows a specific distribution (e.g., an exponential distribution or a uniform distribution).
- *Service discipline*: Service discipline determines the order that patients in a queue. Some commonly used service disciplines in a healthcare service system are first come first served and priority-based.

5.3   Estimating the Performance of Cardiac Surgery Services

We apply the proposed integrated prediction method within the context of the cardiac surgery services in Ontario, Canada, to discover the effects of demographic profiles on cardiac surgery utilization and performance; predict how cardiac surgery utilization and performance change in response to demographic shifts; and demonstrate the dynamics of cardiac surgery performance in terms of queue length and wait times by modeling and simulating the operational process of CS-ORs. The explicit analytical is illustrated in Fig. 5.2.

We introduce the utilized data in Sect. 5.3.1. In Sect. 5.3.2, we describe the hypothetical complex relationships between the *age profile*, *recent immigrant profile*, cardiac surgery *capacity* (i.e., the number of CS-ORs), *supply* (i.e., the number of physicians who are able to perform cardiac surgeries), *service utilization* (i.e., the number of patient arrivals), and performance (i.e., the *throughput* and *wait times* of semi-urgent/elective patients) and test these relationships with SEM. The process of predicting cardiac surgery utilization based on SEM test results is shown in Sect. 5.3.3. The multi-server multi-queue with an entrance control queueing model (MSMQ-EC) used to simulate CS-ORs is shown in Sect. 5.3.4. We present and discuss the estimation and simulation results in Sect. 5.3.5.

5.3.1 Aggregated Data

As described in Sect. 1.4, the aggregated data describing cardiac surgery characteristics and the number of ORs were obtained primarily from the Cardiac Care Network of Ontario (CCN). The aggregated data about physicians for cardiac surgery in each hospital were got from Ontario Physician Human Resources Data Center (OPHRDC). Demographic data on patient age and recent immigration in each local health integration networks (LHIN) were derived from 47 sampled cities and towns (as shown in Fig. 1.4) based on 2006 census data published by Statistics Canada.

In this work, the age profile in an LHIN is defined as the ratio of the population aged 50 years and above to the total population in the LHIN. This age population is of interest because it is the major cohort of cardiac surgery patients [134]. An LHIN's RI profile is the ratio of recent immigrants from Asia and Africa to the total population in the LHIN. We are interested in these ethnic groups because they account for approximately 70% of new immigrants. In addition, prior work has shown that, compared with white groups, the risk factors for cardiovascular diseases are more prevalent in black, South Asian, Southeast Asian, West Asian and Middle Eastern ethnic groups [19, 49]. As patients dwelling in one LHIN may travel to other LHINs to receive cardiac surgeries, we preprocess the demographic data by the cross-LHIN ratio reported by the CCN, so as to more precisely characterize the demographic profiles for each LHIN.

As shown in Fig. 5.2, we used the aggregated data concerning demographic profiles and cardiac surgery characteristics from 2005 to 2007 (12 quarters) as the training data set. The aggregated data from 2008 to 2012 were used to calculate the changes in the demographic profiles and to evaluate the estimated cardiac surgery service utilization and performance. Table 5.1 provides an overview of the training data set.

5.3.2 Relationships Between Demographic Factors and Service Characteristics

We must first derive the hypothetical complex relationships between demographic profiles, cardiac surgery service utilization, and service performance, before the relationships can be tested with SEM. According to prior work, aging and immigration are two major factors accounting for demographic changes [129, 198]. Both *age profile* [13, 19] and *RI profile* [19, 49, 199] may have a positive effect on cardiac surgery *service utilization*. Cardiac surgery *capacity* and *supply* may have effects

Table 5.1 A summarization of the LVs and MVs in the training data set

LV	MV	Mean
Age profile	Ratio of population aged 50 and over in an LHIN	0.34
RI profile	Ratio of recent immigrants from Asia and Africa in an LHIN	0.05
Service utilization	Average number of patient arrivals, monthly	82
Capacity	Number of cardiac surgery physicians, yearly	7
Supply	Number of CS-ORs	3
Throughput	Average number of completed patients, monthly	83
Wait times	Median wait times of S/E patient*	6/19
	Queue length, monthly	58

RI: *profile* recent immigrant profile, *S*: semi-urgent patient, *E*: elective patient, ***: the median wait time of urgent patient is not considered a measurement for the LV wait times because it does not significantly reflect wait times according to our pre-data analysis.

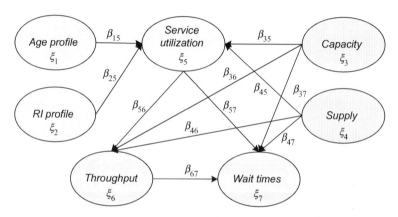

Fig. 5.5 The hypothetical relationships between the demographic profiles, service utilization, and service performance

on *service utilization* [39, 204], *throughput* [44], and *wait times*[44]. *Throughput* may have an effect on *wait times* [44]. We then use the hypothetical relationships to empirically examine the effects of the demographic profiles on cardiac surgery characteristics, as shown in Fig. 5.5. The MVs for each LV in Fig. 5.5 are listed in Table 5.1.

5.3.3   Service Performance Prediction

Once the relationships between the demographic factors and service characteristics have been identified, cardiac surgery performance in response to demographic changes can be predicted by the following sub-steps.

S1: Calculating the values of the exogenous LVs, i.e., the *age profile*, *RI profile*, *capacity*, and *supply*. As the cardiac surgery capacity and supply only change slightly from one year to the next, according to real-world observations, we assume that the cardiac surgery capacity and supply will not change during the estimation time. We can therefore make a clearer observation on how demographic shifts affect cardiac surgery service utilization and performance, and whether existing cardiac surgery resources are capable of providing a stable service in terms of wait times. The changes in the age and RI profiles can be expressed by:

$$\begin{cases} \xi_1 = x_1(1 + \Delta Age)^\tau \\ \xi_2 = x_2(1 + \Delta RI)^\tau, \end{cases} \tag{5.6}$$

where ΔAge and ΔRI are the changes in the age and RI profiles, respectively, at time τ.

S2: Calculating the values of the endogenous LVs, i.e., *service utilization*, *throughput*, and *wait times*, using:

$$\begin{cases} \xi_5 = \beta_{50} + \beta_{15}\xi_1 + \beta_{25}\xi_2 + \beta_{35}\xi_3 + \beta_{45}\xi_4 + \zeta_5 \\ \xi_6 = \beta_{60} + \beta_{36}\xi_3 + \beta_{46}\xi_4 + \beta_{56}\xi_5 + \zeta_6 \\ \xi_7 = \beta_{70} + \beta_{37}\xi_3 + \beta_{47}\xi_4 + \beta_{57}\xi_5 + \beta_{67}\xi_6 + \zeta_7. \end{cases} \tag{5.7}$$

S3: Calculating the values of the MVs that relate to the endogenous LVs, i.e., the number of patient arrivals, queue length, and median wait times for semi-urgent/elective patient. We can therefore estimate the values of cardiac surgery service utilization and performance with respect to changes in the demographic profiles.

5.3.4 The MSMQ-EC Queueing Model

We build an MSMQ-EC queueing model based on the real-life execution of CS-ORs in Ontario, to gain insights into the temporally changing patterns in cardiac surgery performance with respect to demographic shifts. The MSMQ-EC is similar to the queueing model in our prior work [205]:

- M homogeneous ORs with the same service rate μ;
- Three patient groups, urgent (U), semi-urgent (S), and elective (E), with the arrival rates λ_U, λ_S, and λ_E, respectively;
- N physicians maintaining N priority queues.

The service principle of the queueing model is as follows. Urgent patients have the highest priority and should be immediately settled in an available CS-OR. If all of the CS-ORs are occupied, urgent patients must wait and bump the first available CS-OR block for non-urgent patients. Semi-urgent and elective patients are scheduled by physicians following a priority-based service principle. A new incoming non-urgent ($\bar{U}$, i.e., semi-urgent or elective) patient will first be assigned to a physician j ($\forall j \in [1, N]$) with a probability $p_{j,\bar{U}}$. Physician j performs a non-urgent surgery with a probability $q_{j,\bar{U}}$ that represents the "entrance control" of CS-ORs for non-urgent surgeries. Similar to the prior work [205], $p_{j,\bar{U}}$ and $q_{j,\bar{U}}$ follow uniform distributions in the simulation.

5.3.5 Prediction Results

In this subsection, we demonstrate the estimation results of cardiac surgery utilization in the Hamilton Health Science Centre (HHSC) hospital, located in the Hamilton Niagara Haldimand Brant LHIN (LHIN 4), between 2008 and 2011. The complex relationships in cardiac surgery are extracted from the training data set using the software SmartPLS.[1] The simulation results based on the MSMQ-EC queueing model demonstrate the dynamics of cardiac surgery performance. In the simulation, the queueing model was parameterized using the general operational data for the HHSC CS-ORs in 2007. All of the simulation studies are implemented using the discrete-event simulation toolbox SimEvents in MATLAB 2010.

5.3.5.1 The Results of SEM Tests and Service Utilization Estimation

According to the PLS test results (as shown in Fig. 5.6), *service utilization* has an R^2 of 0.631, *throughput* has an R^2 of 0.874, and *wait times* has an R^2 of 0.610. These endogenous LVs are therefore well explained by their dependent variables. For example, the R^2 of the LV *service utilization* reflects that its dependent variables, i.e., *age profile*, *RI profile*, *capacity*, and *supply*, explain 63.1% of the variance in *service utilization*. Although there may be other factors influencing service utilization other than the factors that we have considered, the results imply that the factors used capture most of the variation in service utilization. The PLS test results show that all of the hypothetical effects between the LVs are significant, except the effects of *supply* on *throughput* and *wait times*, and the effect of *throughput* on *wait times*.

It should be noted that LVs with significant correlations (as shown in Fig. 5.6a) can be considered in the prediction process. The path coefficients used in the calculation process are shown in Fig. 5.6b. The *age profile*, *RI profile*, *capacity*, and *supply* should be considered when calculating the value of *service utilization*, as the four exogenous LVs have significant direct effects on *service utilization* according to Fig. 5.6a. Two directly related LVs, *capacity* and *service utilization*, must be

---

[1] www.smartpls.de/. Last accessed on April 11, 2019.

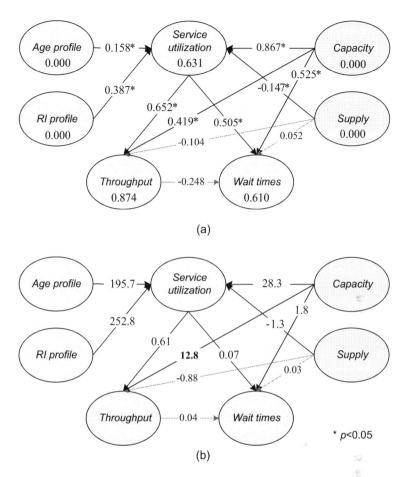

Fig. 5.6 The PLS test results. (**a**) Correlations between the LVs; (**b**) Path coefficients between the LVs. RI recent immigrant

considered when calculating the values of *throughput* and *wait times*, as both of the LVs have significant direct effects. Other LVs, i.e., *age profile*, *RI profile*, *capacity*, and *supply* have significant indirect effects via *service utilization*, so their effects must also be included in the calculation.

The rate of change in the *age profile* in LHIN 4 is 0.073% from 2006 to 2010 and 0.093% from 2006 to 2011 [128], respectively. As detailed information about the *RI profile* in LHIN 4 is not available, we use the trends for Ontario as a whole instead. According to [128], the RI ratio is assumed to be 0.009 of the total population in Ontario since 2008. The estimated cardiac surgery utilization in LHIN 4 is shown in Table 5.2. The estimated results reveal that our method is able to estimate cardiac surgery utilization and wait times to some extent.

Table 5.2 The estimated
values for cardiac surgery
utilization and performance
(average value in a month)

	2010_E	2011_E	2010_A	2011_A
Service utilization	108	115	–	–
Throughput	98	102	83	84
Wait times	14.53	14.98	–	–
Queue length	65	67	–	–
SMW	6.7	7.0	–	–
EMW	20.9	21.6	20	20

E: estimated value in LHIN 4, *A*: actual value in Ontario,
SMW: semi-urgent median wait times, *EMW*: elective
median wait times, –: actual data is not available

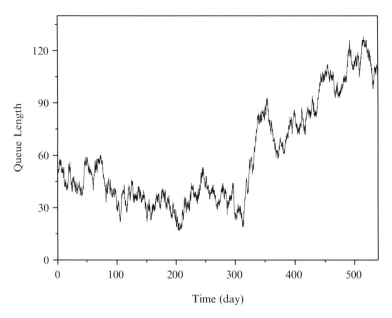

Fig. 5.7 The estimated service utilization and resulting simulated queue lengths from 2010 to
2011

5.3.5.2 Simulation Results Based on the MSMQ-EC Queueing Model

To observe the dynamics of cardiac surgery performance in terms of queue length
and wait times in CS-ORs in 2010 and 2011, we show our simulation results based
on the MSMQ-EC queueing model with the estimated service utilization. According
to the CCN data, we assume that there are 50 patients waiting at the end of 2009.
We initialize the queueing model with three servers (ORs), which can provide 1400
cases annually, in accordance with the actual CS-OR operations in the HHSC. The
simulation results for the queue length and average wait time from 2010 to 2011 are
shown in Figs. 5.7 and 5.8.

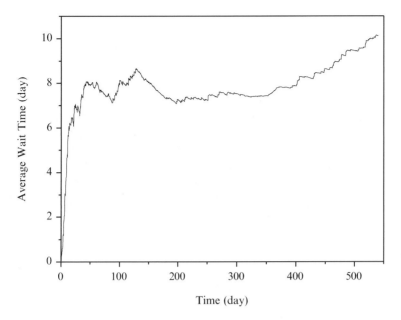

Fig. 5.8 The estimated service utilization and resulting simulated average wait times from 2010 to 2011

5.4 Discussion

The prediction results as shown in Table 5.2 and Figs. 5.7 and 5.8 present the advantages of our integrated prediction methods from two aspects. First of all, according to the estimation results as shown in Table 5.2, the estimated throughput of cardiac surgery services in LHIN 4 is higher than the actual average throughput in Ontario, and the estimated elective wait times for cardiac surgery in LHIN 4 are almost equal to those in Ontario. This finding is in accordance with the observed performance pattern of cardiac surgery services in LHIN 4, as the ratios of the throughput and elective wait times for cardiac surgery in LHIN 4 to those in Ontario are 1.42 and 1.02, respectively, according to the training data set. This reveal that our proposed integrated prediction method is able to identify key impact factors and their complex relationships with service utilization and wait times. Therefore, it is reasonable to predict the service utilization and performance in a middle or long term based on the identified key factors and effects.

Secondly, as shown in Figs. 5.7 and 5.8, our integrated prediction is further able to represent the dynamics of service performance during the prediction period. For instance, according to Table 5.2, the estimated queue lengths in 2010 and 2011 are different. The estimated queue length in 2010 does not increase beyond 60. The pattern does not hold in 2011, in which the simulated queue length shows a sharp increase. The longest queue length reaches 120 in 2011. Higher estimated service utilization in 2011 than in 2010 may account for the rising queue length in 2011, as shown in Fig. 5.7. According to Fig. 5.8, the simulated average waiting time in 2011 is also longer than that in 2010. The average waiting time is around 7 days in 2010 and rises to almost 10 days at the end of 2011.

However, due to the limited data about service utilization and performance, the evaluation of prediction accuracy of the proposed method needs further extension. Possible extensions of this work mainly include two aspect: (1) to give a range of variations in the predicting service utilization and service performance instead of determined values because the assumption that impact factors keep the same changing rate over time is somewhat strong and does not agreement with the real world; (2) to show the deviations of estimated service utilization and performance over time based on queueing model simulations by taking into account the randomness relating to patients' or service providers' behavior.

5.5   Summary

In this chapter, we focused on how to predict the changes in healthcare service performance based on the underlying relationships between the demographic profiles, health service utilization, and service performance. We proposed an integrated prediction method consisting of SEM-based analysis, prediction, and queueing model simulations, and tested the method on cardiac surgery services in Ontario, Canada. The results show that our proposed method can reveal the complex relationships between the demographic profiles and healthcare service characteristics, which enables us to reasonably predict the changes in service utilization and service performance with respect to demographic shifts. Our queueing models, which characterize certain operations within a healthcare service system, allow us to observe the dynamics of the queue length and wait times in response to demographic shifts over time. This method will be helpful for a healthcare service system aiming to dynamically adjust its resources and management strategies, and thus maintain a stable service in terms of performance.

Chapter 6
An Adaptive Strategy for Wait Time Management

Healthcare service managers often consider how to improve service management behavior to better service performance. Commonly-faced problems include how to allocate time blocks of operating rooms (ORs) for patients who have different levels of urgency and how to schedule patients so as to shorten wait times. In this chapter, we discuss how to design adaptive strategies for time block allocations in ORs with the aim of improving service performance with respect to unpredictable patient arrivals. Figure 6.1a summarizes the research focus of this chapter and how it fits into the larger context of understanding a healthcare service system.

The work presented in this chapter shows the method and process of designing and evaluating strategies for improving service management behavior. According to the research steps as shown in Fig. 6.1b, we first propose an adaptive OR time block allocation strategy from a self-organizing systems perspective, which incorporates historical feedback information about ORs. We then evaluate the performance of the proposed strategy using a queueing model derived from general perioperative practices based on discrete-event simulations. This work shows that our proposed adaptive strategy is able to efficiently allocate OR time blocks to deal with unpredictable patient arrivals.

6.1 Introduction

The healthcare service system is a complex system [26, 27] consisting of numerous factors affecting the system's performance, e.g., unpredictable patient arrivals (often referred to service utilization), service capacity, and service management; and interactions (coupling relationships) between the factors and the system's performance/outcome. As one of the major cost areas in hospitals, the operating room (OR) can also be viewed as a typical complex healthcare service system, consisting of a number of impact factors (e.g., unpredictable arrivals) and positive/negative

© Springer Nature Switzerland AG 2019

L. Tao, J. Liu, *Healthcare Service Management*, Health Information Science,
https://doi.org/10.1007/978-3-030-15385-4_6

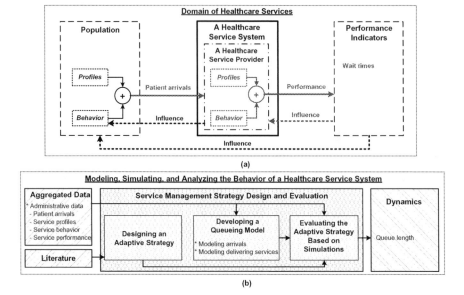

(a)

(b)

Fig. 6.1 A schematic diagram illustrating the design and evaluation of an adaptive strategy for improving time block allocations in ORs. (**a**) The research focus of this chapter (highlighted in red) with respect to the larger context of understanding a healthcare service system. (**b**) Research steps for using the method of service management strategy design and evaluation for OR time block allocations

relationships between those impact factors and OR performance (e.g., the positive effect of arrivals on the waiting time and queue length [44], and the positive effect of service capacity on arrivals [39]). Due to the nature of its complexity, researchers and healthcare administrators have realized that improving the healthcare service system from a self-organizing systems perspective is promising [26, 27]. In this chapter, we aim to improve the utilization of ORs by incorporating an adaptive OR time block allocation strategy proposed from a complex systems point of view.

Different resource management strategies have been proposed to improve the utilization of ORs with respect to different indicators, such as service throughput, average waiting time, queue length, the number of bumped non-urgent surgeries, and the number of unused OR time blocks [206]. A common strategy is to improve the allocation of OR time blocks. Existing studies have attempted to improve OR time block allocation by (1) estimating surgery lengths more accurately (e.g., the time taken to perform a combined coronary artery bypass surgery should be longer than a non-combined case), so that the size of time blocks can be assigned more reasonably [206]; (2) analyzing and controlling the factors that cause surgery delays [207], e.g., reducing the delay of the first surgery to avoid the cancelation of following surgeries in a day, for example; or by (3) strategically arranging non-urgent surgeries, as they account for nearly 85% of all surgeries [208].

A challenging, basic question involved in OR time block allocation is how many OR time blocks should be reserved to cope with the unpredictable arrival of urgent patients. Reserving more time blocks than those are actually needed may cause lower OR utilization, a longer waiting list, and longer wait times for non-urgent surgeries, whereas reserving insufficient time blocks may increase urgent patients' risk, result in more bumped non-urgent surgeries, and prolong the wait times for those bumped cases.

Earlier studies have used mathematical methods (e.g., job shop scheduling models) to compute the optimal number of reserved urgent time blocks. The goal of these methods is to maximize OR time block utilization while minimize the overtime or cancellation of surgeries [56].

In some Ontario hospitals, OR time blocks are distributed to surgeons based on the allocations made in previous years and may only be reviewed two or three times a year. As this allocation strategy is relatively static, it may not cope well with actual patient arrivals. Patient arrivals are dynamic because of the number of impact factors involved, such as the weather and patients' service utilization behavior [19]. Adaptively reserving time blocks in accordance with dynamic patient arrivals will therefore lead to better use of OR resources.

This chapter uses a complex systems perspective to propose an adaptive OR time block allocation strategy for coping with dynamic patient arrivals. We measure the effectiveness of our strategy using the number of bumped non-urgent surgeries (i.e., cancelled surgeries that are replaced by urgent surgeries), and the number of unused urgent time blocks, which are assigned to urgent surgeries in advance but not used. We believe that a more effective OR time block allocation strategy will improve OR utilization. We evaluate the performance of our strategy by building a multi-priority, multi-server, non-preemptive queueing model with an entrance control mechanism based on the general practice of cardiac surgery operating rooms (CS-ORs) in the HHSC[1] in Ontario, and based on which to carry out discrete-event simulations.

6.2 Designing an Adaptive OR Time Block Allocation Strategy

One way to allocate OR time blocks is to reserve a certain number of time blocks for urgent surgeries and assign the remaining time blocks to surgeons for non-urgent surgeries. The number of time blocks allocated for urgent surgeries or to surgeons are usually based on the allocation methods used in previous years [9]. Allocating ORs with such a relatively static strategy may not effectively use ORs as patient arrivals are unpredictable. We therefore propose an adaptive OR time block allocation strategy that incorporates the system's feedback. As illustrated in Fig. 6.2, the main idea behind our strategy is to periodically adjust the time blocks

---

[1]http://www.hhsc.ca/. Last accessed on April 11, 2019.

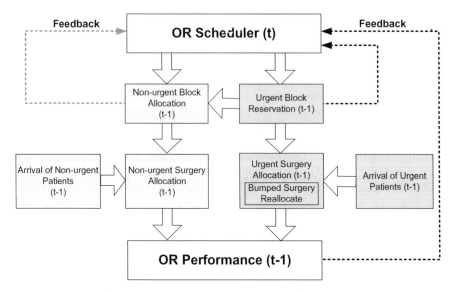

Fig. 6.2 The OR scheduler with a feedback mechanism

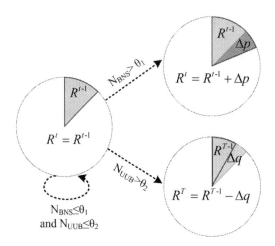

Fig. 6.3 The adjusted window mechanism for updating OR time blocks for urgent surgeries

allocated for urgent surgeries based on the feedback information. In period t, the OR scheduler is fed the OR time block allocation, the numbers of bumped non-urgent surgeries, the unused urgent time blocks, and the dynamic arrivals in $t-1$.

Our adaptive strategy uses an adjusted window mechanism, which is shown in Fig. 6.3. When the OR scheduler makes a decision on the allocation of time blocks for the coming period t, the information from the past period $t-1$ is fed back to the OR scheduler. If the number of bumped non-urgent surgeries is larger than a threshold θ_1 in $t - 1$, the scheduler increases the number of time blocks for urgent surgeries (as denoted as $R(t)$) by a step size of Δp in t. If the number of unused urgent time blocks is larger than a threshold θ_2, the scheduler decreases $R(t)$ by a step size of Δq in T. The thresholds θ_1 and θ_2 are defined by $\theta_i = \frac{b_i * \sigma * t}{\hat{t}}$ ($i \in \{1, 2\}$), where b_i is a positive integer, $\hat{t}$ is a unit of time (1 week here), and σ is the standard threshold in $\hat{t}$.

6.3 Modeling OR Services

We examine the performance of our adaptive strategy by building a queueing model to simulate the queueing situations in ORs with respect to the arrival/service patterns, service discipline (e.g., priority based service discipline), and scheduling strategies. Our queueing model (as shown in Fig. 6.4) is based on the CS-ORs in the Hamilton Health Science Centre (HHSC) in 2004. We assume that there are two homogeneous (in terms of service rate) ORs, each of which has two time blocks in average per day and works 5 days/week. The 1400 patient arrivals for cardiac surgeries each year are categorized into urgent (U), semi-urgent (S), and elective (E) priority groups. According to the historical data from [20], the ratios of U, S, and E patients are 0.23, 0.6, and 0.17, respectively. Patient arrivals in winter are approximately one quarter greater than in other seasons, because of seasonal factors such as weather. We assume that the arrival rate λ_i of each priority group i ($i \in \{U, S, E\}$) follows a Poisson distribution and the service rate μ of each OR follows an Exponential distribution, similar to previous work [96].

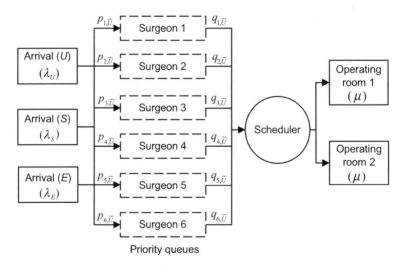

Fig. 6.4 A multi-priority, multi-server, non-preemptive queueing model with an entrance control mechanism

According to the scheduling rule, U patients are settled immediately in an available OR as they have the highest priority. If all of the ORs are unavailable, U patients bump the first prescheduled OR block for non-urgent surgery. In reality, a number of OR time blocks are reserved to cope with U patients. In our model, we use δ_0 to denote the initial number of time blocks reserved for urgent surgeries in a unit of time $\hat{t}$ ($\hat{t} = 1$ week in this work). S and E patients are scheduled by surgeons following a priority-based service principle. New non-urgent (i.e., S and E) patients are assigned to a surgeon j ($j \in [1, 6]$ in our case denotes one of the six surgeons) with a probability $p_{j,\bar{U}}$ ($\bar{U}$ denotes non-urgent patients) and then wait in the queue of surgeon j. In reality, surgeons normally perform non-urgent surgeries in time blocks allocated to them in advance. Therefore, we assume that a patient at the head of a queue j will move to the OR with a probability $q_{j,\bar{U}}$ at the next time step. It should be noted that $p_{j,\bar{U}}$ and $q_{j,\bar{U}}$ follow uniform distributions in our simulations.

The queueing model is implemented using the discrete-event simulation toolbox SimEvents integrated with MATLAB 2010. The parameters in the simulations are initialized with statistical data from the HHSC in 2004. The performance of the adaptive strategy and its sensitivity to the parameter settings are investigated in specific scenarios.

6.4 Simulation-Based Experiments

6.4.1 Aggregated Data and Experimental Settings

HHSC is one of the most comprehensive healthcare service systems in Ontario, Canada. Approximately 1400 cardiac surgeries are performed each year in this hospital. In 2004, it had six specialized surgeons and two ORs. The aggregated data about the operations of HHSC come from several organizations. Reports published by the Surgical Process Analysis and Improvement Expert Panel in Ontario[2] and by the Office of the Auditor General of Ontario Hospitals [9] list the general rules for scheduling ORs in the HHSC. The data representing the performance of the HHSC since 2004, including the number of surgeries completed in each month (throughput) and the number of patients waiting at the end of each month (queue length) also come from CCN. Furthermore, a study in collaboration with the HHSC in 2004 [206] reported data on the average service time per surgery and the number of canceled surgeries. Table 6.1 summarizes the HHSC cardiac surgery data, which are utilized to initialize our simulations.

---

[2]http://www.health.gov.on.ca/en/pro/programs/ecfa/quality/research/cst_periop.aspx. Last accessed on April 11, 2019.

Table 6.1 Cardiac surgery services in the HHSC in 2004

Performance indicator	Data
Queue length (at the end of a month)	
Quarter 1	156
Quarter 2	159
Quarter 3	149
Quarter 4	147
Cancellations	
Bumped non-urgent surgeries	77
Service time	
Average	4.6 h

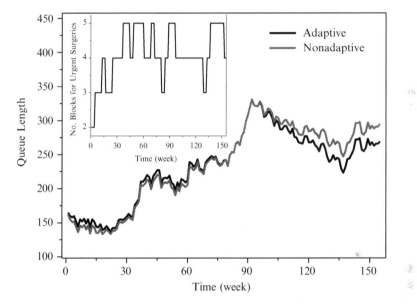

Fig. 6.5 The simulated queue lengths over 3 years. Inserted plots: the time blocks for urgent surgeries allocated with the adaptive strategy. Settings: $\delta_0 = 7$/week, $\hat{t} = 4$ weeks, $\theta_1 = 2 * \hat{t}$, $\theta_2 = 1 * \hat{t}$, $\Delta p = 1$, $\Delta q = 1$

6.4.2   Experimental Results

We first investigate the effect of our adaptive strategy in shortening queue lengths over a 3-year period (i.e., 156 weeks, where 13 weeks represents one quarter in the simulation and the third quarter each year corresponds to the winter season) using the queueing model. As shown in Fig. 6.5, the average queue length with the adaptive strategy is slightly shorter than that without the adaptive strategy. Please note that simulation results are obtained from a single simulation run with patient arrival patterns described in the preceding section and parameter settings as given in the figure caption. Queue lengths at the initial time step ($t = 0$) in the simulation are both set to 156, which is the number of patients who were waiting for cardiac surgeries at the end of 2003 in HHSC. The fluctuations in queue lengths, especially the increasing periods in the weeks 27–39, 79–91, and 131–143, correspond to the increased patient arrivals in the winter compared with other seasons.

The existing OR time block allocation strategy depends heavily on the allocation methods used in previous years. A hidden assumption behind this strategy is that patient arrivals do not vary much within a year. This assumption may not hold in reality as patient arrivals are dynamic in response to the complex environment (e.g., the weather) and patients' personal behavior. The static time block allocation strategy may therefore result in a number of bumped non-urgent surgeries when there are more urgent arrivals, or it may lead to under-utilization of OR time blocks due to fewer urgent arrivals. The strategy proposed in this chapter adaptively adjusts OR time blocks based on historical information, for example, the utilization of ORs in the previous week/month/quarter and the number of urgent/non-urgent arrivals.

6.5   Discussion

We conduct several additional simulation experiments with different parameter settings (i.e., the initial reserved blocks for urgent surgeries in a week, the adjustment time interval, threshold, and step size) to confirm the observations made. Figure 6.6 shows that without the adaptive strategy, the number of bumped non-

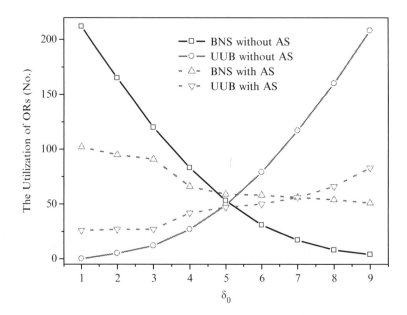

Fig. 6.6 OR utilization with respect to different initial urgent OR time blocks. AS adaptive strategy, BNS bumped non-urgent surgeries, UUB unused urgent time blocks, $\delta_0 = 7/$week, $\hat{t} = 4$ weeks, $\theta_1 = 2 * \hat{t}, \theta_2 = 1 * \hat{t}, \Delta p =, \Delta q = 1$

urgent surgeries drops and the number of unused time blocks increases when δ_0 increases. This finding suggests that the utilization of ORs without the adaptive strategy is more sensitive to the number of time blocks allocated to urgent surgeries, whereas the adaptive strategy is robust to the initial number of OR blocks for urgent surgeries. The figure also shows that the OR can maintain a trade-off between the number of bumped non-urgent surgeries and the number of unused urgent time blocks with the adaptive strategy. This finding implies that hospitals can adapt to dynamically changing patient arrivals with our adaptive strategy and hence can improve their OR utilization. Furthermore, Fig. 6.6 reveals that OR utilization is improved when δ_0 is set to 5–8.

The time interval T for allocating OR time blocks (e.g., once per week/month/quarter) is another key parameter in the adaptive strategy. Figure 6.7 shows the effects of different updating time intervals (i.e., a unit of time $\hat{t}$) on OR utilization in terms of the trade-offs between the numbers of bumped non-urgent surgeries (BNSs) and unused urgent time blocks (UUB). We measure the trade-off with $\frac{N_{BNS}}{N_{UUB}}$, where N_{BNS} denotes the number of BNS and N_{UUB} represents the number of UUB. OR utilization improves as the value of the trade-off approaches 1 (represented by the dotted line in Fig. 6.7). As Fig. 6.7 shows, updating the OR time block once every 4–8 weeks will both reduce the number of bumped non-urgent surgeries and balance the number of unused urgent blocks. In the scenario as presented in this figure, updating the OR time block once every 4 weeks will result in the best OR utilization.

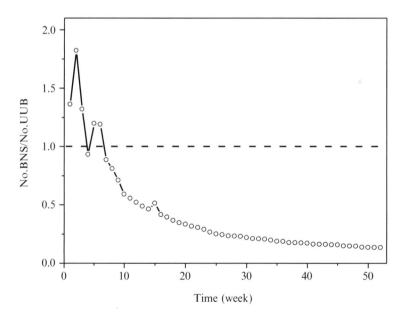

Fig. 6.7 The trade-offs ($\frac{N_{BNS}}{N_{UUB}}$) of the adaptive strategy with respect to different $\hat{t}$. Settings: $\delta_0 = 7/\text{week}$, $\theta_1 = 2 * \hat{t}$, $\theta_2 = 1 * \hat{t}$, $\Delta p = \Delta q = 1$

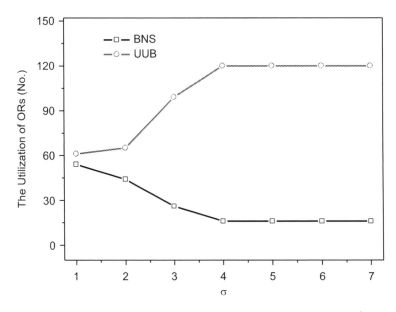

Fig. 6.8 OR utilization with respect to adjustment thresholds. Settings: $\delta_0 = 7/\text{week}$, $\hat{\imath} = 4\,\text{weeks}$, $\theta_1 = 2 * \sigma * \hat{\imath}$, $\theta_2 = \sigma * \hat{\imath}$, $\Delta p = \Delta q = 1$

The adjustment thresholds (θ_1 and θ_2) and the step sizes (Δp and Δq) may also affect the performance of the adaptive strategy. According to Fig. 6.8, larger adjustment thresholds (i.e., larger σ) result in a larger number of unused urgent time blocks and a smaller number of bumped non-urgent surgeries. This is reasonable, as seven time blocks are initially reserved for urgent surgeries, which almost satisfy the average number of urgent arrivals in a week according to the patient arrival patterns. Intuitively, larger thresholds make ORs less likely to increase or decrease the time blocks for urgent surgeries, and vice versa. In such cases, the adaptive strategy will be less flexible and hence can lead to a worse OR utilization.

Figure 6.9 shows that smaller step sizes (e.g., Δp and Δq are set to 1 or 2) can guarantee better OR utilization in the given specific scenario. Intuitively, a larger step size will lead to the number of time blocks for urgent surgeries increasing or decreasing by a larger amount at a time, and thus will result in a larger number of unused urgent time blocks or bumped non-urgent surgeries in the next time step.

We can fine-tune the parameter settings of the adaptive strategy using the above results. Figure 6.10 presents a comparison of the queue lengths generated by the original adaptive strategy (defined by Setting I, which is the same as the setting configuration of the adaptive strategy in Fig. 6.5), the fine-tuned adaptive strategy (defined by Setting II), and by the allocation schedule without the adaptive strategy. The fine-tuned adaptive strategy has a shorter queue length than the original adaptive strategy most of the time.

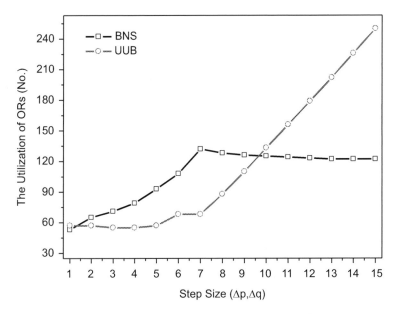

Fig. 6.9 OR utilization with respect to step sizes. Settings: $\delta_0 = 7/\text{week}$, $\hat{t} = 4\,\text{weeks}$, $\theta_1 = 2 * \hat{t}$, $\theta_2 = \hat{t}$

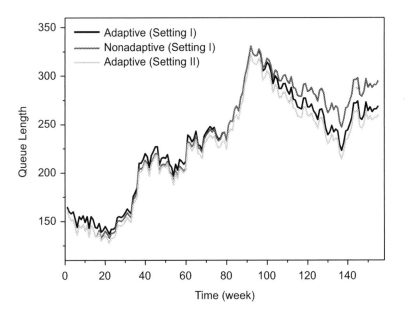

Fig. 6.10 Queue lengths generated by different block allocation strategies. Setting I: $\delta_0 = 7/\text{week}$, $\hat{t} = 4\,\text{weeks}$, $\theta_1 = 2*\hat{t}$, $\theta_2 = 1*\hat{t}$, $\Delta p = \Delta q = 1$; Setting II: $\delta_0 = 5/\text{week}$, $\hat{t} = 4\,\text{weeks}$, $\theta_1 = 2*\hat{t}$, $\theta_2 = 1 * \hat{t}$, $\Delta p = \Delta q = 1$

6.6   Summary

In this chapter, we proposed an adaptive strategy for allocating OR time blocks based on a feedback mechanism. We evaluated the effectiveness of the adaptive strategy in improving the utilization of service resources using a specific multi-priority, multi-server, non-preemptive queueing model with an entrance control mechanism based on the general perioperative process of CS-ORs. Simulation results showed that our adaptive strategy is able to efficiently regulate OR time block reservations in response to the dynamics of patient arrivals. The adaptive strategy could maintain a better trade-off between the number of bumped non-urgent surgeries and the number of unused urgent OR time blocks, leading to shorter waiting lists and wait times. The findings presented in this chapter suggest that frequently adjusting the OR time block allocation (i.e., once per month) is helpful for improving OR utilization. The work shown in this chapter also demonstrates that the method of service management strategy design and evaluation from a complex systems perspective is promising for improving service management.

Chapter 7
Spatio-Temporal Patterns in Patient Arrivals and Wait Times

When regional healthcare service managers review the operations of healthcare services in a past period of time, they often feel confused about some of the unexpected spatio-temporal patterns in patient arrivals and wait times. How did these patterns emerge? What reasons and mechanisms account for the emerging patterns? How can patient arrivals be regulated at different hospitals and thus improve the service utilization in the region? In this chapter, we present how to use our proposed behavior-based autonomy-oriented modeling method to characterize the spatio-temporal patterns in cardiac surgery services in Ontario, Canada, with the aim of answering some of the aforementioned questions. Figure 7.1a summarizes the research focus of this chapter with respect to the larger context of understanding a healthcare service system and the corresponding research steps.

The work shown in this chapter presents the process of using the behavior-based autonomy-oriented modeling method to characterize emergent spatio-temporal patterns at a systems level by taking into account the underlying entities' behavior (e.g., the patients' hospital selection behavior) with respect to various impact factors (e.g., the distance between homes and services, hospital resourcefulness, and historical wait time information). According to the steps of the behavior-based autonomy-oriented modeling method shown in Fig. 6.1b, we first develop an Autonomy-Oriented Computing (AOC)-based cardiac surgery service model (AOC-CSS model). By experimenting with the AOC-CSS model, we reveal the working mechanisms that explain how the spatio-temporal patterns in patient arrivals and wait times at a systems level emerge from individual patients' hospital selection behavior and their interactions with hospital wait times. The work presented in this chapter also reveals that our proposed behavior-based autonomy-oriented modeling method is useful in finding the underlying reasons for emergent spatio-temporal patterns in complex healthcare systems.

© Springer Nature Switzerland AG 2019
L. Tao, J. Liu, *Healthcare Service Management*, Health Information Science,
https://doi.org/10.1007/978-3-030-15385-4_7

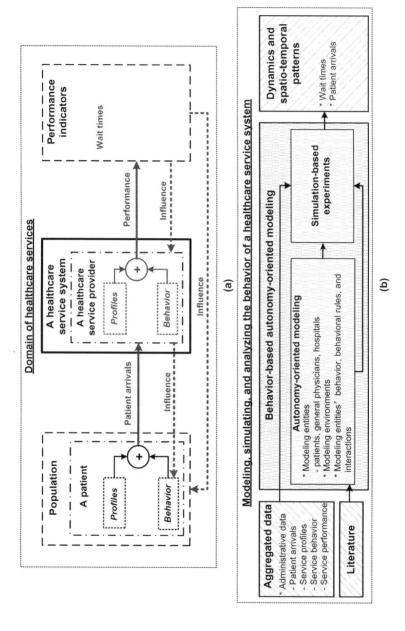

Fig. 7.1 A schematic diagram illustrating the use of the behavior-based autonomy-oriented modeling method to characterize the emergent spatio-temporal patterns in patient arrivals and wait times in a healthcare service system. (**a**) The research focus of this chapter (highlighted in red) with respect to the larger context of understanding a healthcare service system. (**b**) Research steps for using a behavior-based autonomy-oriented modeling method to analyze the behavior of a healthcare service system

7.1 Introduction

A healthcare service system, such as the cardiac care system schematically illustrated in Fig. 7.2, is well recognized as a complex system [26, 27]. Some interesting self-organizing spatio-temporal patterns in healthcare service utilization, such as the power-law distribution of variations in the time that patients spend on specialists' waiting lists [39], have been reported. However, it is still unclear what individual behavior and underlying factors (e.g., distance from homes to services, hospital resourcefulness in terms of physician supply, and service performance) account for these emergent spatio-temporal patterns.

In this chapter, we use a behavior-based autonomy-oriented modeling method to understand some spatio-temporal patterns relating patient arrivals and wait times from a complex systems self-organizing perspective within the context of cardiac surgery services. To model the real-world cardiac surgery system in Ontario, Canada, the following essential issues must be addressed.

- *Scope*: What factors, entities, processes, and hierarchical levels (e.g., services at a hospital or regional level) are relevant to the spatio-temporal patterns, and hence should be investigated and modeled?
- *Coupling relationships and/or interactions*: What are the relationships between the impact factors and variables? What local feedback loop(s) is(are) crucial for understanding global-level self-organized regularities and thus should be modeled?
- *Heterogeneity*: Patient behavior when choosing a hospital may be heterogeneous due to the differences in personal profiles, and service distributions in and around their residence areas. Hospitals may also be heterogeneous in delivering healthcare services because of variations in equipped resources and management strategies. Thus, capturing the heterogeneity of patients and hospitals is essential in modeling a real-world healthcare service system.

We use a behavior-based autonomy-oriented modeling method [36] to construct an AOC-CSS model. In modeling the real-world cardiac care system in Ontario, Canada, we consider multiple factors affecting patient arrivals (as shown in Fig. 7.2), such as weather, demographics of cities and towns in Ontario, geographic accessibility of cardiac surgery services, resourcefulness of a hospital, wait times, and patients' hospital selection behavior.

Following a behavior-based autonomy-oriented modeling method, we firstly introduce the spatio-temporal patterns in patient arrivals and wait times, which are observed from the aggregated data on cardiac surgery services. We then identify the key entities, major factors, and local feedback loops that should be modeled. After that, we present the detailed formulation of the developed AOC-CSS model, along with model-based simulations and corresponding results. We finally discuss the underlying mechanism that is revealed by the validated AOC-CSS model and a sensitivity analysis on the key parameters that influence the emergence of self-organized patterns.

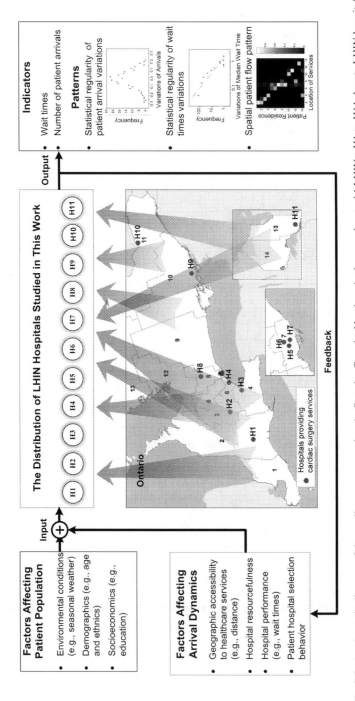

Fig. 7.2 A schematic diagram of the cardiac surgery services in Ontario, Canada. Numbers in the map denote 14 LHINs. H1 to H11 denote LHIN hospitals. The spatio-temporal patterns on the right-hand side are examples to show those observed from secondary data about cardiac surgery service utilization between January 2005 and December 2006

7.2 Empirical Spatio-Temporal Patterns in Cardiac Surgery Services

Prior studies have empirically identified self-organized regularities in healthcare systems. For instance, Smethurst and Williams found that the monthly absolute variations in the time that patients spend on specialists' waiting lists (calculated as the change in the mean wait times $\bar{w}$ at time steps t and $t - 1$ $(\bar{w}_t - \bar{w}_{t-1})/\bar{w}_t$) followed a power-law distribution [39] and concluded that hospital waiting lists were self-regulating. We aim to discover the corresponding patterns in the cardiac surgery services from empirical data, focusing on three research questions.

1. What are the statistical distributions of the variations in the number of patient arrivals and wait times?
2. What are the spatial patterns of patient flows? Are there any underlying patterns that may be observed from the spatial distribution of patient flows?
3. What are the temporal patterns in patient arrivals and wait times?

We once again focus on the cardiac care system in the province of Ontario, Canada, specifically the Ontario Local Health Integration Networks (LHINs). The Cardiac Care Network of Ontario (CCN) has published monthly wait time information for cardiac surgery services in 11 member hospitals across Ontario between January 2005 to December 2006. We accessed the data in February 2011. As shown in Table 4.1, the reported CCN data include the number of completed cases in a month (i.e., throughput), the average number of patients waiting at the end of a month (i.e., queue length), and the monthly median wait times for urgent, semi-urgent, and elective patients. We use the median wait times for elective patients (referred to hereafter as the median wait times) to measure wait times, which represents the changes in the overall wait times for cardiac surgery services to a great extent.

Based on the CCN data, we are able to calculate the average monthly number of patient arrivals at each hospital by:

$$A_i(t) = B_i(t) + Q_i(t) - Q_i(t - 1), \tag{7.1}$$

where $A_i(t)$ is the average monthly number of arrivals in quarter t of unit i, $B_i(t)$ is the average monthly number of patients who have received treatment in quarter t of unit i, and $Q_i(t)$ is the average number of patients waiting at the end of a month in quarter t of unit i.

We use the above-described data for cardiac surgery services over 2 years, from January 2005 to December 2006, to discover the self-organized patterns in patient arrivals and wait times.

7.2.1   Statistical Regularities

Following the work of Smethurst and Williams [35, 39], we first investigate the statistical distributions of the variations in patient arrivals and wait times. From the CCN data, the month-to-month variations in patient arrivals and wait times are calculated by:

$$v_{t+1} = \frac{y_{t+1} - y_{min}}{y_{max} - y_{min}} - \frac{y_t - y_{min}}{y_{max} - x_{min}}, \tag{7.2}$$

where v_{t+1} denotes the variation in patient arrivals or wait times at time $t + 1$, y_t denotes the number of patient arrivals or the wait times at time t, y_{min} and y_{max} are the minimum and the maximum values of patient arrivals or wait times over the 2-year period, respectively. In this work, each time step t corresponds to a month.

The absolute month-to-month variations in patient arrivals or wait times, v'_t, are then calculated by:

$$v'_t = |v_t|. \tag{7.3}$$

Two types of self-organized regularities are identified from the (absolute) variations in patient arrivals and wait times, as shown in Figs. 7.3 and 7.4. As shown in Fig. 7.3, the monthly variations in patient arrivals against the percentage of variation occurrences follow a normal distribution with a mean value of 0.004 and a standard deviation (SD) of 0.226. The normality of the distribution passes the Kolmogorov-Smirnov test [209, pp. 392–394].

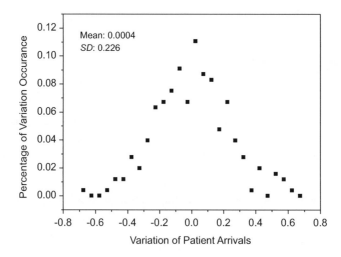

Fig. 7.3 The statistical distribution of variations in patient arrivals for cardiac surgery services in Ontario, Canada, between January 2005 and December 2006

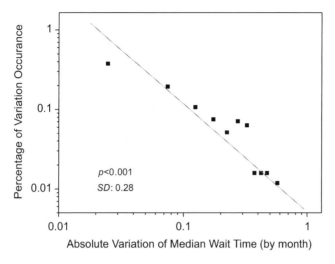

Fig. 7.4 The statistical distribution of the absolute variations in median wait times for cardiac surgery services in Ontario, Canada, between January 2005 and December 2006

As shown in Fig. 7.4, the monthly absolute variations in the median wait times follow a power-law distribution with a power of -1.36 and a standard deviation of 0.28 (linear fitness: $p < 0.001$). The fitness of the power-law distribution is tested using the method proposed by Clauset et al. [210] (power-law test: $p < 0.1$). The median wait times for cardiac surgery services therefore exhibits a statistical regularity in its month-to-month variations, suggesting that the cardiac care system is, to a degree, able to self-organize [211] its wait times.

7.2.2 Spatial Patterns

7.2.2.1 Patient Flow Distributions

Figure 7.5 shows the distribution of the number of patients residing in each LHIN against the LHINs where they receive cardiac surgery services between 2007 and 2008 in Ontario, Canada [136]. The distribution can be regarded as the spatial pattern of patient flows, which represents the aggregated effects of patients' hospital selection behavior. We find approximately the same spatial pattern using the reported statistical data from 2007 to 2011 [69, 136, 212–214]. The percentage of cardiac surgery patients operated in an LHIN with respect to their LHIN residence varies within 5% year to year over the 4 years, with a maximum value of approximately 10%.

Fig. 7.5 The distribution of cardiac surgery patients with respect to their LHIN residences between 2007 and 2008 in Ontario, Canada

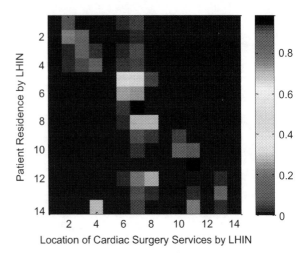

Location of Cardiac Surgery Services by LHIN

7.2.2.2   Patient-Attraction and Patient-Distribution Degrees for LHINs

The spatial pattern of patient flows shown in Fig. 7.5 may represent additional information about the probability that an LHIN attracts patients residing in other LHINs, called the patient-attraction degree, or the probability that patients living in a specific LHIN travel to other LHINs for services, called the patient-distribution degree. A higher patient-attraction degree indicates that the LHIN is linked by more patients from other LHINs and reveals how heavily patients from other LHINs can affect the arrivals for the hospital(s) in a specific LHIN. A higher patient-distribution degree indicates that patients living in that LHIN are more likely to disperse to other LHINs to receive cardiac surgery services. This in turn reveals the extent to which patients in a specific LHIN may influence arrivals at hospitals in other LHINs. In this section, we introduce how to reveal this underlying information and the corresponding patterns.

Calculation Method
We use the idea behind the hyperlink-induced topic search (HITS) algorithm designed by Kleinberg [215] to calculate the patient-attraction degree and the patient-distribution degree for each LHIN from the patient flow distribution. The HITS algorithm is a linkage structure-based analysis algorithm. It characterizes to what extent a web page is an "authority" by estimating the in-degree of a page, or to what extent it is a "hub" by estimating the out-degree of a page, based on the relationships between a set of related web pages.

Our method is similar to the HITS algorithm. Based on the distribution of patient flows, LHINs can form a network structure where a directed link between two LHINs indicates that there are patients coming from the LHIN the link points away from, to the LHIN the link points toward. Thus, an LHIN can be regarded as analogous to a web page, its patient-attraction degree as analogous to the "authority" value of a web page, and its patient-distribution degree as analogous to the "hub" value of a web page. We can therefore estimate the values of the patient-attraction degree and patient-distribution degree for each LHIN via the eigenvectors of the matrices associated with the distribution of patient flows, as proposed by Kleinberg [215].

Given a patient-flow matrix $P_F = \{f_{ij}\}_{N \times M}$, each entry f_{ij} of F is the percentage of patients residing in LHIN i and receiving cardiac surgery services in LHIN j. Based on Kleinberg's theorem [215, p. 11], the patient-attraction degree vector (i.e., the authority weight vector in the HITS algorithm) is the principle eigenvector of $P_F^T P_F$ and the patient-distribution degree vector (i.e., the hub weight vector in the HITS algorithm) is the principle eigenvector of $P_F P_F^T$. We use the patient flow distribution between 2007 and 2008, using data obtained from [136], to calculate the patient-attraction degree and the patient-distribution degree for each LHIN.

Patient-Attraction and Patient-Distribution Degrees
We calculate the patient-distribution degree and the patient-attraction degree for each LHIN using the method described above. From the patient-distribution degrees shown in Fig. 7.6, we observe that LHINs can be roughly classified into two groups, a high-patient-distribution group and a low-patient-distribution group. LHINs in the high-distributed group (LHINs 5–9 and 12) have obviously larger distributed degrees than those in the low-distributed group (LHINs 1–4, 10, 11, 13, and 14). These two distributed groups may be related to the geographic accessibility to services (service accessibility) for each LHIN. The LHINs in the high-distributed group are more accessible to cardiac surgery services than the LHINs in the low-distributed group, according to the service accessibilities presented in Table 3.1.

From the patient-attraction degree for each LHIN shown in Fig. 7.6, we again observe that the LHINs can be roughly classified into two groups, a high-patient-

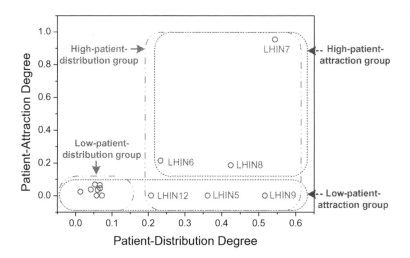

Fig. 7.6 The distribution of LHINs' patient-attraction and patient-distribution degrees

attraction group and a low-patient-attraction group. The LHINs in the high-patient-attraction group (LHINs 6–8) have more patients traveling from other LHINs than the LHINs in the low-patient-attraction group (LHINs 1–5 and 9–14). The formation of the two groups may be driven by the geographic locations and reputations (e.g., the number of physicians and wait times) of the hospitals in each LHIN. For instance, LHIN 7 has the highest patient-attraction degree and is the only LHIN with three hospitals, which all have sufficient personnel and facilities. LHIN 6 and 8's relatively higher patient-attraction degrees could be because these LHINs have hospitals providing cardiac surgeries and they have one or more neighboring LHINs that lack cardiac surgery services (e.g., LHIN 5, 9, and 12), as shown in Fig. 1.3.

7.2.3 Temporal Patterns

As patient arrivals and wait times change dynamically, there may be temporal regularities, in addition to the statistical and spatial patterns already identified. We aim to identify any existing temporal patterns, focusing on two specific research questions.

1. What are the changing trends in patient arrivals and wait times? Are there any patterns in the temporal variations in patient arrivals and wait times, such as monthly or seasonal patterns?
2. As historical information about the wait times in each hospital is expected to affect the subsequent patient arrivals, does the cardiac care system exhibit patterns that reveal the potential interactions between patient arrivals and wait times?

Figures 7.7 and 7.8 show the monthly variations in patient arrivals and wait times, respectively, in cardiac surgery services in Ontario from 2005 to 2006. Although patient arrivals for cardiac surgery services fluctuate from month to month in both Ontario (shown in Fig. 7.7a) and in each hospital (shown in Fig. 7.7b), there is a seasonal pattern. Cardiac surgery services have relatively smaller numbers of patient arrivals in the warm season (shown as the shadowed areas in Fig. 7.7a), which runs from the fifth month (May) to the eighth month (August), than in the colder months.

We observe a similar seasonal pattern in the dynamically changing wait times in Fig. 7.8. The median wait times in Ontario consistently decrease from the sixth month (June) to the tenth month (October) each year, shadowed in Fig. 7.8. The lower wait times may be due to the lower patient numbers in cardiac surgery services in the warm season, as illustrated in Fig. 7.7a.

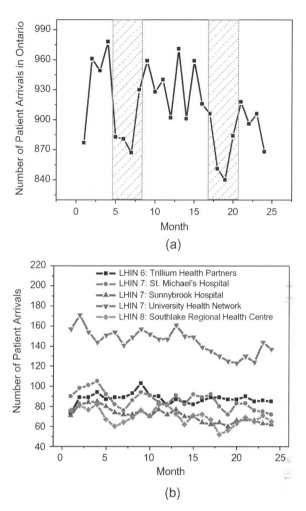

Fig. 7.7 The changes in patient arrivals for cardiac surgery services in (**a**) Ontario, and (**b**) five hospitals that provide cardiac surgery services

7.3   AOC-CSS Modeling

7.3.1   Identifying Key Elements in Modeling

7.3.1.1   Entities

In Ontario, each location (e.g., a city or a town) has a certain number of patients that require cardiac surgery services. When these patients are recommended to have cardiac surgeries by their general practitioners (GPs) or specialists, they will choose a specific hospital to receive the required services from [216]. In most cases, patients make their decisions with their GPs, as 93% of Ontario's population are registered with a GP [217] and most of the patients will follow a GP's

Fig. 7.8 The changes in the median wait times for cardiac surgery services in (**a**) Ontario, and (**b**) five hospitals that provide cardiac surgery services

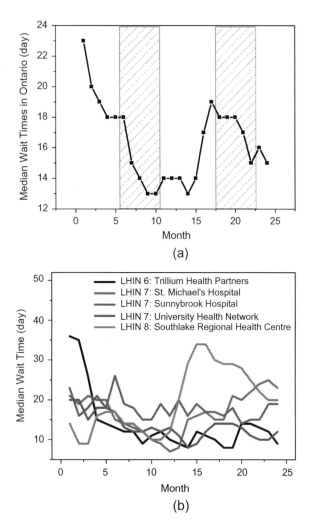

recommendations [28, 218]. Patient hospital selection behavior therefore represents the consequence of a patient-GP mutual decision. After patients make a decision on hospital selection, they visit the selected hospital and wait to receive the treatment [216]. Finally, patients leave the hospital after finishing the treatment. From the afore described process, we can therefore identify three entities in the cardiac care system, the *patient*, the *GP*, and the *hospital*.

7.3.1.2 Major Impact Factors

Dynamically changing patient arrivals and wait times may be directly or indirectly affected by various factors. These factors, as illustrated in Fig. 7.2, can be divided into two categories.

- Factors affecting the patient population: Factors such as environment (e.g., weather), demographics (e.g., population size and age), and socioeconomics (e.g., education), may affect the number of patients who have cardiovascular disease. Thus, we consider these factors when initializing the parameter of generating patient population for each city or town in simulations.
- Factors affecting the dynamics of patient arrivals to hospitals: Factors such as the geographic distance between homes to a hospital, hospital reputation (e.g., hospital resourcefulness), hospital performance (e.g., wait times), and decision making style may affect patients' hospital selection behavior, and thus result in the variations of patient arrivals to each hospital. We therefore consider these factors when designing behavioral rules for patients and hospitals.

In our modeling, based on the literature and our SEM-based studies (please refer to Chaps. 3 and 4 for these studies), the factors that affect the patient population and thus should be considered in the simulation initialization are summarized below.

- *Geodemographic profile of a location*: As we investigated in Chap. 3, cities and towns with distinct geodemographic factors have different patient arrivals for cardiac surgery services. We therefore consider the differences in the geodemographic profiles of locations, which are represented by the patient arrival rate in the modeling.
- *Seasonal weather*: Seasonal weather is an important contributing factor for the outbreak of many diseases, including cardiac diseases [19], and therefore influences patient arrivals and wait times in cardiac care services. For instance, as shown in Fig. 7.5, the patient arrival rate in the warm season (from May to October) in Ontario is approximately 15% lower than that in the cold season (from January to April and from November to December), according to the reported CCN data [136]. We therefore consider the factor of seasonal weather in our modeling, which is represented in different arrival rates in warm and cold seasons.

The identified major factors that influence the patient behavior in selecting hospitals and the hospital behavior in delivering services and thus are considered in our modeling are summarized below.

- *Geographic distance*: As revealed by our SEM-based analysis (please refer to Chap. 3 for the study) and the literature, the geographic distance between homes and a hospital is negatively associated with the probability that patients and GPs select a hospital [11, 219], because patients are more likely to visit hospitals close to their homes. Thus, we take into account the geographic distance in modeling patients' hospital selection behavior.

- *Hospital resourcefulness*: The resourcefulness of a hospital, represented by the number of physicians [29] in this study, is positively correlated with the probability that patients and GPs select a specific hospital [29, 220, 221] because more hospital resources may attract more patient arrivals [39]. We therefore consider this factor when designing behavioral rules for patients' hospital selection behavior.
- *Hospital performance* in terms of wait times: Wait times for receiving the required cardiac care services are a major concern for patients [28] and GPs [11, 222], who are usually in favor of hospitals with short wait times [11, 28, 222]. We therefore take this factor into consideration when designing behavioral rules for patients.

7.3.1.3   Local Feedback Loops

The impact factors of wait times may have complex relationships, coupled interactions, and/or feedback loops [57]. These interactions, especially the local feedback loops, may result in nonlinear phenomena (e.g., self-regulating patient arrivals and wait times) in the complex cardiac care system.

We identify two local feedback loops between the impact factors, shown in Fig. 7.9. The first negative feedback loop (namely AW-loop) exists between the factors of patient arrivals and wait times, due to the patient-GP mutual decisions on hospital selection. For instance, long wait times in a hospital may weaken the probability of patients and GPs selecting that hospital, which will in turn decrease the number of patient arrivals and result in a decrease in wait times.

As shown in Fig. 7.9, the factors of patient arrivals, hospital service rate, and wait times form a positive feedback loop (named as ASW-loop) due to hospitals' service

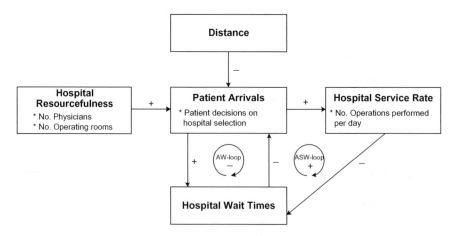

Fig. 7.9 The effects of impact factors on patient-GP mutual decisions on hospital selection and the local feedback loops. +/−: a positive or negative relationship between two factors

adjustment behavior. If there are more patient arrivals at a hospital, that hospital will increase its service rate. Wait times will therefore decrease, which will in turn result in a larger number of patient arrivals.

7.3.2 Modeling Environment

In this study, the geographic relationship/structure between patients' locations and hospitals is conceptualized as a bipartite location-hospital network CH, defined below.

Definition 7.1 (Location-Hospital Network) A location-hospital network can be described as a bipartite network $CH = (C, H, F, I)$. The location node set $C(N) = \{c_i\}$ ($i \in [1, N]$) denotes N cities, towns, or concerned sub-regions as patients' locations. The hospital node set $H(M) = \{h_j\}$ ($j \in [1, M]$) represents M hospitals that provide specific healthcare services, $H \cap C = \emptyset$. The adjacent matrix $F = \{f_{ij}\}_{N \times M}$ ($f_{ij} \in [0, 1]$, $\sum_{j \in [1, M]} f_{ij} = 1$) represents whether or not there are patient flows between each pair of city-hospital nodes. $IN = \{in_{ij}\}_{N \times M}$ represents the static or dynamic information between each pair of city-hospital nodes.

Here, each location node c_i ($\forall c_i \in C$) represents a city or town with a population of more than 40,000 in 2006 in Ontario, Canada, according to census data. Each hospital node h_j ($\forall h_j \in H$) denotes a hospital that provides cardiac surgery services in Ontario, Canada. The location-hospital information is defined as $IN = \{in_{ij}(t) | i \in [1, N], j \in [1, M]\} = \{d_{ij} | i \in [1, N], j \in [1, M]\}$, where d_{ij} represents the distance from a city or town c_i ($\forall c_i \in C$) to a hospital h_j ($\forall h_j \in H$). Following Chap. 3, the distance d_{ij} is represented by the driving time between a city or town and a hospital. The driving time is again estimated using the "Get directions" function in Google Maps.

Based on the location-hospital network CH, the environment E in the AOC-CSS model records the released information about hospitals. We formally define the environment E as described below.

Definition 7.2 (Environment) The environment E for the AOC-CSS model is represented by a bipartite network, as defined in Definition 7.1. E maintains information that can be accessed by patients and GPs. We define the environment E as a tuple $< D, RS, W >$, where the elements are defined as follows:

- D: Distance information $D = \{d_{ij} | i \in [1, N], j \in [1, M]\}$. Each d_{ij} records the driving time between a city/town c_i ($\forall c_i \in C$) and a hospital h_j ($\forall h_j \in H$).
- RS: Hospital resourcefulness information $RS = \{rs_j | j \in [1, M]\}$, where rs_j records the number of physicians in h_j ($\forall h_j \in H$).
- W: Wait time information $W = \{w_{j,\tau} | j \in [1, M]\}$. Each $w_{j,\tau}$ records the wait time information for a hospital h_j ($\forall h_j \in H$) at time round τ. Here, a unit time round τ to review hospital operations (e.g., 1 month or one quarter) includes NT number of unit time steps t (a unit of time to record the hospital operational

information, e.g., 1 day), i.e., $\tau = NT * t$. In this paper, $w_{j,\tau}$ records the median wait times of h_j over the past time round $\tau - 1$.

7.3.3   Modeling Entities

7.3.3.1   Patient

As reported in [28], a large number of patients may not have access to wait time information and thus they may not consider wait times when they select a hospital. Patients can therefore be categorized as *wait time-sensitive* or *wait time-insensitive*, according to their decision making styles. *Wait time-sensitive* patients consider all of the acquired information about the hospitals (i.e., distance, hospital resourcefulness, and wait times). *Wait time-insensitive* patients do not take in to account wait time information when they select hospitals. A patient entity is defined as described below.

Definition 7.3 (Patient Entity) A patient entity, *patient*, maintains a record: $< patientID, cityID, P_r, rule, hospitalID, type, joinTime, endTime, \tilde{w} >$, where the elements are defined as follows:

- *patientID*: This records the unique identity represented by a constant for a patient.
- *cityID*: This denotes the unique identity for the city/town that a patient comes from.
- P_r: This denotes the probability of a patient considering the factor of wait times when selecting a hospital. Accordingly, the probability of a patient who does not take into account the factor of wait times when choosing a hospital is $1 - P_r$.
- *rule*: This indicates how a patient chooses a hospital along with the GP.
- *hospitalID*: This indicates the unique identity for the hospital that a patient arrives at.
- *type*: This represents the urgency of a patient entity to the cardiac surgery service according to the severity of illness, $\forall k \in [1, K]$ ($K \geq 1$). In this study, there are two urgent types: urgent patients and non-urgent patients.
- *joinTime*: This denotes the time step that a patient joins in the queue of a hospital.
- *endTime*: This indicates the time step that a patient has been served in a hospital.
- $\tilde{w}$: This records the wait time information of a patient, $\tilde{w} = endTime - joinTime$.

7.3.3.2 GP

In the AOC-CSS model, patients come to a hospital that is selected by patient-GP mutual decisions and the released information in the environment E. As most cardiac surgery patients are referred by GPs, we define entities $GP[N]$ to record and represent patient-GP mutual decisions on hospital selection, as described below.

Definition 7.4 (GP Entity) $GP[N]$ records the information about patients who live in specific locations and receive cardiac surgery services. Each entity GP_i ($i \in [1, N]$) maintains a record: $< cityID, A_k(t) >$, where the elements are defined as follows:

- $cityID$: This represents the unique identity of a location.
- $A_k(t)$: This denotes the patient flow information for urgent type k ($k \in K$) patients, $A_k(t) = \{\hat{a}_{k,j}(t)\}$. Each $\hat{a}_{k,j}(t)$ records the number of type k ($k \in K$) patients to hospital h_j ($h_j \in H$) at time step t.

7.3.3.3 Hospital

We model the operations of a hospital entity based on queuing theory. As CS-ORs in a hospital are, to a certain extent, homogeneous, it is reasonable to regard a hospital j as one server (i.e., one OR) with a service rate μ_j, and thus assume that each hospital is an M/M/1 queuing model [223]. A hospital entity is defined as described below.

Definition 7.5 (Hospital Entity) $Hospital[M]$ records the information on all of the hospitals. Each hospital entity h_j ($\forall h_j \in H$) maintains a record $< hospitalID, cityID, \tilde{A}_k(t), \mu(t), rule, w(\tau), Q >$, where the elements are defined as follows:

- $hospitalID$: This represents the unique identity for a hospital.
- $cityID$: This indicates the unique identity for the city/town in which a hospital is located.
- $\tilde{A}_k(t)$: This records the patient arrival information for type k ($k \in K$) patients, $\tilde{A}_k(t) = \{\tilde{a}_{i,k}(t)\}$. Each $\tilde{a}_{i,k}(t)$ records the number of type k ($k \in K$) patients coming from city/town c_i at each time step.
- $\mu(t)$: This denotes the hospital service rate at time step t.
- $rule$: This represents how the hospital adjust the service rate with respect to the accumulated patient arrivals. The specific rule will be formally described in the next subsection.
- $w(\tau)$: This records the wait time information of hospital h_j in a past time period, which will be released in environment E. In this work, the wait time information w released at time round τ is the average median wait times for the past time round $\tau - 1$.
- Q: This records the information about the queue that includes all the patient entities waiting for cardiac surgery services at each time step.

7.3.4 Designing Behavioral Rules

7.3.4.1 Behavioral Rules for Patients Selecting Hospitals

Based on the literature review and the analysis of variable relationships presented in Chaps. 3 and 4, we identify stylized facts regarding the effects of key factors that influence patient-GP mutual decisions for hospital selection and the variations of patient arrivals in hospitals.

- *Stylized fact 1*: The probability that patients select a hospital is exponentially and inversely related to the distance between their homes and a hospital [21].
- *Stylized fact 2*: Patients usually prefer to visit a hospital that is resourceful in terms of personnel (e.g., physicians) and facilities (e.g., ORs) [29, 220, 221]. Hospital resourcefulness and the number of patient arrivals are therefore positively correlated [44].
- *Stylized fact 3*: Patients usually prefer to visit a hospital with shorter wait times [11, 28, 222]. However, a large proportion of patients, especially the elderly, may not have access to wait time information or are less likely to consider the wait times when they select hospitals [28].

Based on the stylized facts, we develop two specific behavioral rules, i.e., a DHW rule and a DH rule, to model how patients choose a hospital. The two behavioral rules are our assumptions in this work, which are defined below.

Definition 7.6 (DHW Rule) DHW stands for distance, hospital resourcefulness, and wait times. This rule represents how a patient residing in the location c_i ($\forall c_i \in C$) estimates the arrival probability a_{ij} for a hospital h_j ($\forall h_j \in H$), using the distance d_{ij}, hospital resourcefulness rs_j, and released wait time information $w_j(\tau)$ at time τ. The hospital selection probability for a hospital h_j is calculated by:

$$a_{ij} = f(d_{ij}) * f(r_j) * f(w_j(\tau))$$

$$f(d_{ij}) = \frac{d'_{ij}}{\sum_{h_k \in H} d'_{ik}}$$

$$d'_{ij} = \frac{\sum_{h_k \in H} d_{ik}^{\alpha_d}}{d_{ij}^{\alpha_d}} \qquad (7.4)$$

$$f(r_j) = \frac{r_j^{\alpha_r}}{\sum_{h_k \in H} r_k^{\alpha_r}}$$

$$f(w_j(\tau)) = \frac{\sum_{h_k \in H} w_j^{\alpha_w}(\tau)}{w_j^{\alpha_w}(\tau)},$$

where α_d ($\alpha_d \in [0, 1]$), α_r ($\alpha_r \in [0, 1]$), and α_w ($\alpha_w \in [0, 1]$) are exponential parameters indicating the sensitivity of patients to the factors of distance, hospital resourcefulness, and wait times, respectively.

Definition 7.7 (DH Rule) DH stands for distance and hospital resourcefulness. This rule represents how a patient chooses a hospital h_j with respect to the distance d_{ij} and hospital resourcefulness rs_j. The hospital selection probability is calculated by:

$$a_{ij} = f(d_{ij}) * f(r_j)$$

$$f(d_{ij}) = \frac{d'_{ij}}{\sum_{h_k \in H} d'_{ik}}$$

$$d'_{ij} = \frac{\sum_{h_k \in H} d^{\alpha_d}_{ik}}{d^{\alpha_d}_{ij}} \quad (7.5)$$

$$f(r_j) = \frac{r^{\alpha_r}_j}{\sum_{h_k \in H} r^{\alpha_r}_k}.$$

7.3.4.2   A Behavioral Rule for Hospitals to Adjust Their Service Rates

Hospitals may periodically change their service rates to adapt to unpredictable patient arrivals. For instance, as shown in Fig. 7.10, changes in the throughput,

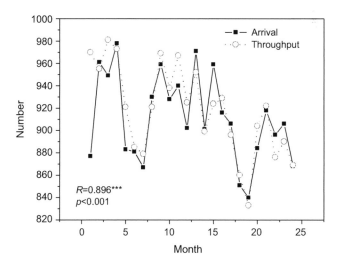

Fig. 7.10 The number of patient arrivals versus the number of treated cases in the cardiac surgery service in Ontario, Canada, between January 2005 and December 2006

which represents the actual serviced numbers of patients, follows approximately the same pattern as changes in the patient arrivals in cardiac surgery services in Ontario. The correlation coefficient between the throughput and patient arrivals is 0.896 ($p < 0.0001$), implying that the service rate of a hospital may vary in accordance with the changes in patient arrivals. We therefore define an S rule for hospitals to adjust their service rates by assuming that service rate of a hospital and the queue length (representing the accumulated patient arrivals at present) is positively and linearly related. The definition of the S rule is given as below.

Definition 7.8 (S Rule) S stands for service rate adjustment. This rule represents how a hospital h_j ($\forall h_j \in H$) changes its service rate $\mu_j(\tilde{T})$ in response to the aggregated patient arrivals at the past time $\tilde{T} - 1$. The service rate adjustment is calculated by:

$$\mu_j(\tilde{T}) = \bar{\mu}_j * (\frac{a_j * A_j(\tilde{T} - 1)}{\bar{A}_j} + b_j), \tag{7.6}$$

where $\tilde{T}$ is the frequency that hospitals adjust their service rate (usually 1 week in Ontario [9]); $\mu_j(\tilde{T})$ is the service rate of a hospital h_j at time $\tilde{T}$; $\bar{\mu}_j$ is the average service rate of a hospital h_j; $A_j(\tilde{T} - 1)$ is the aggregated patient arrivals at the time $\tilde{T} - 1$; $\bar{A}_j$ is the average patient arrivals at a hospital h_j; and a_j and b_j are two adjustment parameters.

7.4   Simulation-Based Experiments

In this section, we conduct simulations based on our AOC-CSS model, aiming to understand the observed spatio-temporal patterns in wait times in the cardiac care services.

7.4.1   Experimental Settings

The parameters in the AOC-CSS model are initialized using publicly available data. The CCN published monthly statistical reports on cardiac surgery service utilization in Ontario hospitals between January 2005 and December 2006. The average number of treated cases, the median wait times, and the queue length in a month for each hospital are reported. Therefore, the service rate μ_j for a hospital h_j can be approximated as the average number of served cases in a day. The arrival rate for each patient type in the city/town c_i can be approximated by:

$$\sum_{k \in K} G P_i . \lambda_k = s_i * m_i, \tag{7.7}$$

where s_i is the patient-generation probability, i.e., the probability that a person in the city/town c_i is a patient who needs a cardiac surgery service, and m_i is the size of the total population in the city/town c_i. The parameter s_i represents the heterogeneity of the city/town c_i in producing a patient population requiring cardiac surgery services with respect to its demographics and socioeconomic factors. The patient-generation probabilities for the cities and towns in each LHIN can be inferred from [20]. The total population m_i for each city/town is gathered from the 2006 Canada Census data.[1]

As seasonal weather is an important contributing factor influencing patient arrivals [19], the arrival rate is adjusted seasonally in our simulation. The patient arrival rate is approximately 15% lower in the warm season (from May to October in Ontario) than in the cold season (from January to April and from November to December in Ontario), according to the reported CCN data.

Near 20% of patients consider wait times when they select hospitals [28]. Therefore, we assume that the probability that a patient considers the factor of wait times when selecting a hospital is relatively small and we set this probability $P_r = 0.2$ in our simulations.

According to the practice, patients are categorized into two types, urgent and non-urgent, i.e., $K = 2$. Following the data reported in [20, p. 71], the arrival rate of urgent patients versus that of non-urgent patients is set to 0.23:0.77. Urgent patients have a higher priority for receiving cardiac surgery services than non-urgent patients.

The values of the exponential parameters (α_d, α_r, and α_w) are estimated using the spatial pattern of real patient flows (shown in Fig. 7.5). Based on our experiments, we found that the mean and standard deviation of absolute errors have relatively small values when $\alpha_d = 4$, $\alpha_r = 1$, and $\alpha_w = 1$. Here, the absolute error is defined as $|e_{ij}| = |\hat{a}_{ij} - \hat{a}'_{ij}|$, where e_{ij} is the error between the actual percentage of patients residing in LHIN l_i who attend hospitals in LHIN l_j from 2007 to 2008 in Ontario (as denoted as $\hat{a}_{ij}$), and that obtained from our simulations (as denoted as $\hat{a}'_{ij}$).

We run our simulations over 2 years, so that the simulated data can be directly compared to the observed real-world data. At each time step, the simulation runs 1000 times and generates an average number of patient for each city/town.

7.4.2 Statistical Regularities in Patient Arrivals and Wait Times

In this section, we examine the statistical regularities in patient arrivals and wait times in our synthetic cardiac care system. Figure 7.11 compares the distribution of the variations in patient arrivals in the real world (represented by the squares in the figure) and the distribution obtained from the simulation (represented by the stars in

---

[1]http://www12.statcan.gc.ca/census-recensement/2006/index-eng.cfm. Last accessed on April 11, 2019.

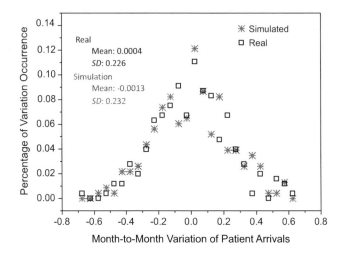

Fig. 7.11 The distributions of variations in simulated and observed patient arrivals in cardiac surgery services

the figure). The simulation approximately reproduces the shape of the distribution of observed patient-arrival variations, shown in Fig. 7.11. The observed patient-arrival variations have a mean of 0.0004 and a standard deviation of 0.226, whereas the simulated patient-arrival variations have a mean of 0.0013 and a standard deviation of 0.232.

The relative entropy or the Kullback-Leibler (KL) divergence is a measure of the difference between two probability distributions [224]. The KL divergence of the statistical distribution of simulated patient-arrival variations from that of real-world patient-arrival variations is 0.1398. The small value of the KL divergence implies that the distribution of patient-arrival variations obtained from the simulation may approximate that of the real world.

Figure 7.12 presents the statistical distribution of absolute variations in the median wait times obtained from our simulation. The absolute variations in the median wait times follow a power-law distribution with a power of -1.47 (linear fitness: $p < 0.0001$). The fitness of the power-law distribution is tested using the Clauset method [210] (power-law test: $p < 0.1$). This distribution indicates that the synthetic cardiac surgery service is self-organizing in terms of its wait times.

Figure 7.13 compares the statistical distribution of absolute variations in the median wait times obtained from our simulation to the distribution of the observed data. The KL divergence of the distribution of the simulated absolute wait-time variations (represented by stars in the figure) from that of the observed absolute wait-time variations (represented by squares in the figure) is 0.1227. The small value of the KL divergence implies that the two distributions are similar.

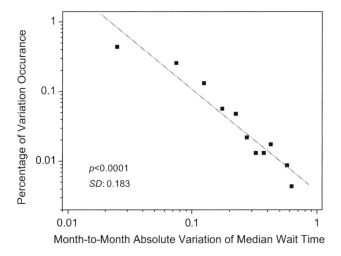

Fig. 7.12 The distribution of simulated absolute wait times variations (by month) in cardiac surgery services

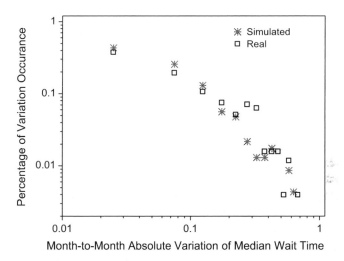

Fig. 7.13 The distributions of simulated and observed wait times variations in cardiac surgery services

7.4.3 Patient-Attraction and Patient-Distribution Degrees of LHINs

Figure 7.14 compares the observed and simulated distributions of LHINs' patient-attraction degrees and patient-distribution degrees. The simulated patient-attraction and patient-distribution degrees for each LHIN are approximately the same as the observed degrees, except for LHIN 12, which has a lower simulated patient-

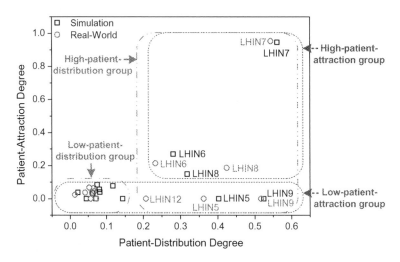

Fig. 7.14 A comparison of the simulated and observed distributions of LHINs' patient-attraction and patient-distribution degrees

distribution degree than that observed in the real world. In the simulation, most patients living in LHIN 12 select the hospital in LHIN 8 because it has the shortest driving time (0.6 h). However, in the real world, although LHIN 6 and 7 are not next to LHIN 12 and have longer driving times (1.2 h and 1.1 h, respectively), approximately 25% of patients who live in LHIN 12 visit the four hospitals (Trillium Health Parters, St. Michael's Hospital, Sunnybrook Health Sciences Centre, and University Health Network) in LHIN 6 and 7, as these hospitals have good resources and the driving time between homes and these hospitals are short enough to be acceptable.

The simulated distributions in Fig. 7.14 exhibit low- and high-patient-attraction groups, and low- and high-patient-distribution groups that are almost the same as the groups exhibited by the observed distributions, shown in Fig. 7.6. LHINs 5–9 have obviously larger patient-distribution degrees and thus form a high-patient-distribution group, whereas LHINs 1–4 and 10–13 have less patients travelling to other LHINs for cardiac surgery services and thus fall into the low-patient-distribution group. Similarly to the observed distributions, LHINs 6–8 exhibit higher attraction degrees in the simulation and thus form a high-patient-attraction group, whereas the other LHINs (LHINs 1–5 and 9–14) fall into the low-patient-attraction group.

7.4.4   Spatio-Temporal Patterns in Patient Arrivals and Wait Times

7.4.4.1   The Dynamics of Patient Arrivals in Each Hospital

Figures 7.15 and 7.16 compare the observed and simulated temporal patterns in patient arrivals for each hospital and show that our AOC-CSS model is able to approximately reproduce the observed temporal patterns in patient arrivals, as the

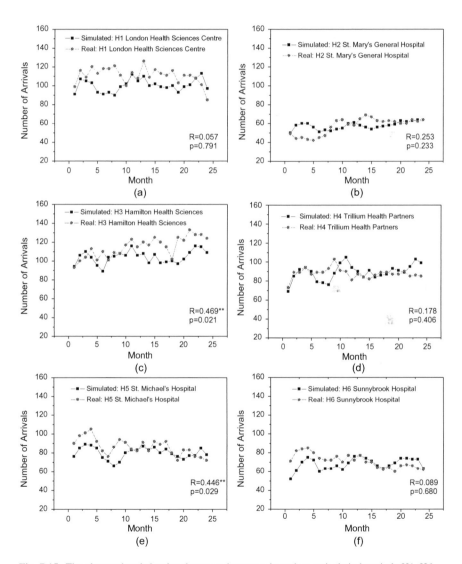

Fig. 7.15 The observed and simulated temporal patterns in patient arrivals in hospitals H1–H6

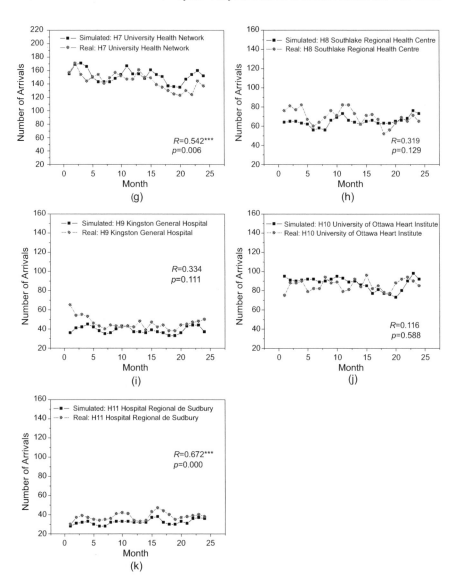

Fig. 7.16 The observed and simulated temporal patterns in patient arrivals in hospitals H7–H11

correlation coefficient R of the simulated and observed patient arrival variations for each hospital is positive.

7.4.4.2   The Dynamics of Wait Times in Each Hospital

Figures 7.17 and 7.18 compare the observed and simulated temporal patterns of the median wait times for each hospital and show that our AOC-CSS model is able to

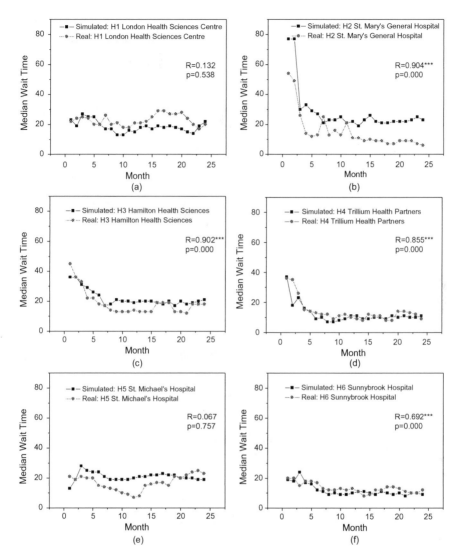

Fig. 7.17 The observed and simulated temporal patterns in wait times in hospitals H1–H6

approximately reproduce the observed temporal pattern of median wait times, as the correlation coefficient R of the simulated and observed patient arrival variations for each hospital is positive.

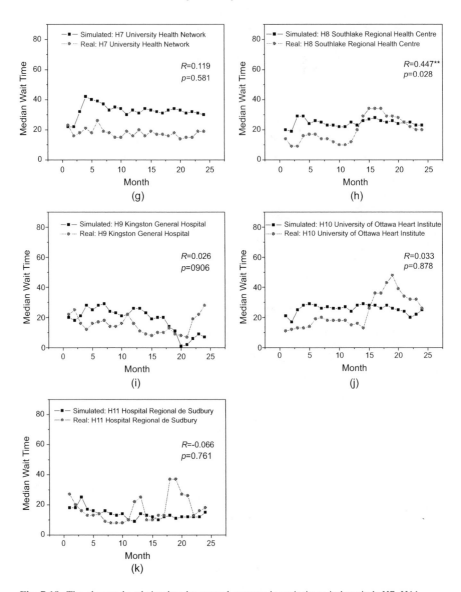

Fig. 7.18 The observed and simulated temporal patterns in wait times in hospitals H7–H11

7.5 Discussion

7.5.1 Explaining the Underlying Causes of Spatio-Temporal Patterns

Based on our AOC-CSS model and simulation-based experiments, we are able to characterize the spatio-temporal patterns in patient arrivals and wait times as observed in real-world cardiac surgery services. These patterns are partially due to the local feedback loop between patient arrivals and hospital wait times, shown in Fig. 7.9.

Let us take the city of Brampton, Ontario, as an example to illustrate the self-organizing process at an individual level. The four hospitals which are nearest to Brampton and offer cardiac surgery services are Trillium Health Parters (H4), St. Michael's Hospital (H5), Sunnybrook Hospital (H6), and University Health Network (H7). The average driving times for patients living in Brampton to travel to these hospitals are less than 0.7 h. Figure 7.19 presents the dynamically changing preferences of patients residing in Brampton for the four hospitals and shows that patients living in Brampton generally prefer H7, because the driving distances from

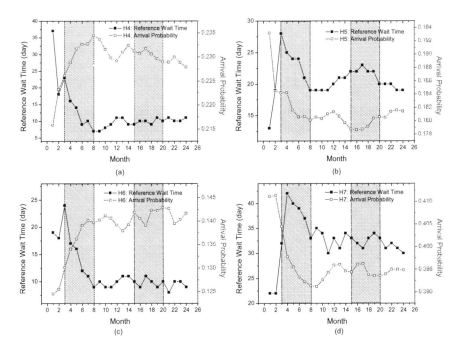

Fig. 7.19 The dynamically changing preferences of patients residing in the city of Brampton (in LHIN 5) to the four neighboring hospitals. (**a**): H4, Trillium Health Partners; (**b**): H5, St. Michael's Hospital; (**c**): H6, Sunnybrook Hospital; (**d**): H7, University Health Network. The shaded areas in this figure represent the warm seasons in Ontario, Canada

Brampton to the four hospitals are almost the same, varying between 0.5 h and 0.7 h, and H7 has more physicians than the other three hospitals. As the values for the factors of driving distance and hospital resourcefulness are not changed during the simulation, the changing wait times for the four hospital are the only cause of the dynamically changing arrival probabilities.

For instance, Fig. 7.19d shows that in the first 2 months, the arrival probabilities for patients living in Brampton for H7 are high, because the wait times in this hospital are short, at approximately 22 days. Due to the high arrival probabilities in the first 2 months, more patients may prefer to visit H7 than the other three hospitals, which will in turn result in longer wait times in H7. The wait time information for H7 is then released into the environment and is used by patients when they make hospital selection decisions in the third month. As a result, the arrival probability of patients living in Brampton for H7 in the third month will decrease. This self-regulating process is initiated by autonomous patient/GP entities according to their hospital selection behavioral rules and incorporates the feedback loop between wait times and hospital selection behavior, potentially accounting for the observed self-organized spatio-temporal patterns at a systems level.

Figure 7.19 also shows that the trends of the changes in arrival probabilities for the four hospitals are complementary. The increase in arrival probabilities to some of the hospitals in some months therefore accompanies the decrease in arrival probabilities to other hospitals. Due to the differences in the wait times in the four hospitals, a few patients may therefore transfer between the four hospitals to avoid a long wait. For instance, in the first warm season (from month 3 to month 8), the arrival probabilities for H4 and H6 increase because their reference wait times are less than 20 days, whereas the arrival probabilities for H5 and H7 decrease because their wait times are much longer than 20 days. It should be noted that although the arrival probabilities for H4 and H6 increase, the wait times in all four hospitals decrease in the first warm season. The number of patient arrivals in the warm season is smaller than in the cold season. As more patients may be willing to travel to H4 and H6 in the first warm season, the accumulated patient arrivals in the first warm season may result in the increase in wait times in the initial several months in the second cold season (from month 9 to month 12), which will in turn reduce the arrival probabilities for the two hospitals. With the same analysis process described above, we can explain the variations in the arrival probabilities and wait times for the four hospitals in the subsequent months.

7.5.2 Sensitivity Analysis

To investigate the sensitivity of our results, we now discuss the statistical distributions of the median wait times with respect to different time scales for calculating the variations in wait times; and different probabilities (i.e., P_r) that a patient takes the wait time information into account when making hospital selection decisions.

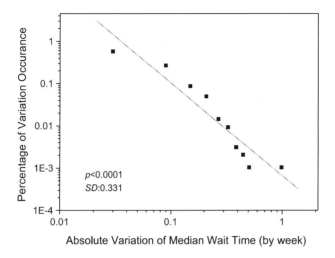

Fig. 7.20 The distribution of simulated absolute wait times variations (calculated by week) in cardiac surgery services

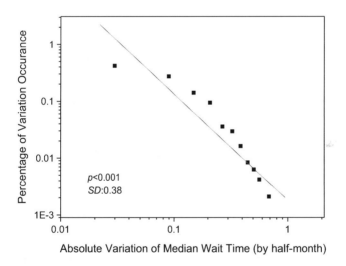

Fig. 7.21 The distribution of simulated absolute wait times variations (calculated by half-month) in cardiac surgery services. The distribution follows a power law with a power of -1.86 ($p < 0.1$; linear fitness (red line, $p < 0.001$; standard deviation $SD = 0.38$)

7.5.2.1 Wait Times Variations at Different Time Scales

Figures 7.20 and 7.21 show the statistical distributions of absolute wait times variations calculated by week and by half-month, respectively. We use the method developed by Clauset et al. [210] to test whether our simulated data follows a power law distribution. We find that the absolute wait times variations presented in the two

figures both fit a power-law distribution (power-law test: $p < 0.1$). The power of
the statistical distribution calculated by week is -2.19 and calculated by half-month
is -1.86, suggesting that absolute wait times variations in different time scales are
able to represent the self-organizing property of the cardiac care system in terms of
wait times, such as by week (as shown in Fig. 7.20), by half-month (as shown in
Fig. 7.21), and by month (as shown in Fig. 7.12).

7.5.2.2   The Probability for Selecting DHW Rule, P_r

Figure 7.22 shows the distributions of absolute wait times variations (calculated
by month) in cardiac surgery services with respect to different probabilities that
a patient considers wait times when choosing a hospital, P_r. Table 7.1 presents
the corresponding p-values of power-law tests with respect to various P_r based
on Clauset's method [210]. According to Fig. 7.22 and Table 7.1, when there are
no wait time-sensitive patients (i.e., $P_r = 0$) who take into account the wait
time information when choosing hospitals, the distribution of absolute wait times
variations does not follow a power-law distribution, as the power-law test is not
significant ($p = 0.13$). If all of the patients select hospitals without considering

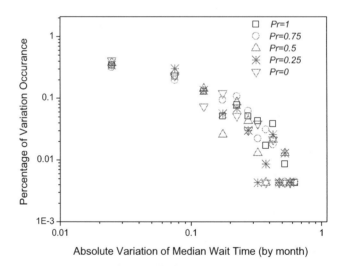

Fig. 7.22 The distributions of absolute wait times variations (by month) in cardiac surgery
services with respect to different P_r

Table 7.1 The p-values of power-law tests for distributions of absolute wait times variations with
respect to different P_r

P_r	1	0.75	0.5	0.25	0
p-value	0.16	0.16	0.16	0.10	0.13

the wait time information, the feedback loop between the patient hospital selection behavior and wait times is absent. Thus, patient arrivals cannot adapt to the dynamically changing wait times in hospitals.

According to Fig. 7.22 and Table 7.1, when there is a relatively small probability that a patient considers wait times when choosing a hospital, e.g., $P_r = 0.25$, the distribution of absolute variations in the median wait times follows a power-law distribution (as suggested by Clauset et al. [210], if $p \leq 0.1$, the data for the power-law fitness test follows a power-law distribution). This suggests that the system is self-regulating due to the wait time-sensitive patients who select different hospitals in accordance with the variations in wait times in each hospital.

However, when P_r becomes large, for instance, 0.5, 0.75, or 1, as shown in Fig. 7.22 and Table 7.1, the distributions of absolute wait time variations do not follow power-law distributions. The p-values of the power-law tests are all larger than 0.1. A large number of wait time-sensitive patients may therefore not result in a self-regulating healthcare service system, as the patient arrivals for each hospital may fluctuate highly if more patients are sensitive to the wait time information when they select hospitals. This can be observed in Fig. 7.22, which shows that larger P_r values result in larger variations in absolute wait time variations.

7.5.3 Remarks on Future Extensions

The work presented in this chapter can be extended from several directions. First of all, the proposed AOC-CSS model does not take into account how opinions and experiences of socially connected people affect patients' hospital selection decisions. The model also omits the topological structure between interacting doctors and patients. However, in the real world, prior patients' experiences with specific service providers and physicians may spread through a social network, and thus affect the hospital selection decisions of subsequent patients. The influence of socially connected people, which is referred to as social influence in the literature, plays a significant role in patients' choice of hospitals [225]. It therefore would be valuable to extend the current AOC-CSS model by incorporating the effects of social influence and by taking into account the various social structures between patients and doctors. By doing so, we may thus develop a more realistic model for characterizing patients' hospital selection behavior. The extended model may also enable us to evaluate the effects of patients' experience and social interactions on the emergent spatio-temporal patterns in service utilization and wait times.

Secondly, this work assumes that all physicians in hospitals are homogeneous in serving patients. Based on this assumption, specific queuing models have been developed to characterize the behavior of hospitals. As physicians may differ in how they prioritize and serve patients [202], the allocated time blocks for serving patients [226], and their medical skills [226], future research could take into account the heterogeneity in physicians. The resulting extended hospital models may better represent the actual operation of healthcare services. Furthermore, modeling heterogeneous physicians may help to design more practical strategies for improving service management behavior.

Finally, in the current work as presented in this chapter, we have investigated how patients select hospitals with respect to the factors of distance, resourcefulness, and wait times, which are identified as key impact factors based on the SEM-based analysis and the literature review. However, the perceived hospital reputation, an unobserved factor that covers patients' perceptions of multiple dimensions, such as hospital resourcefulness, physicians' medical skill, and service outcome, is another important factor influencing patients' choices of a hospital [38, 227]. In the future work, it would be interesting for us to consider the perceived hospital reputation into our AOC-CSS model, so as to better represent the real-world situations and evaluate the effects of hospital reputation on the dynamics of patient arrivals to different hospitals.

7.6 Summary

In this chapter, we used a behavior-based autonomy-oriented modeling method to characterize the spatio-temporal patterns in a cardiac care system from a complex self-organizing systems perspective. We described three types of entities, patients, GPs, and hospitals, and the environment that they reside in and access information from. Based on the identified major impact factors of distance, hospital resourceful-ness, and wait times, and their interaction relationships and local feedback loops, we derived specific behavioral rules for wait time-sensitive and wait time-insensitive patients to make mutual decisions with their GPs on hospital selection. We also designed a specific behavioral rule for hospitals to adjust their service rates with respect to the waiting patients. Through simulation-based experiments, we observed that the constructed white-box AOC-CSS model produces spatio-temporal patterns that are approximately similar to those observed in the real-world cardiac surgery system. The patient-GP mutual hospital selection behavior and its relationship with hospital wait times may therefore account for self-regulating service utilization. The study also revealed that the behavior-based autonomy-oriented modeling method provides a potentially effective means for explaining the self-organized regularities and investigating emergent phenomena in complex healthcare systems.

Chapter 8
An Intelligent Healthcare Decision Support System

In the previous chapters, we showed how to systematically utilize the four specific methods, i.e., *Structural Equation Modeling (SEM)-based analysis*, *integrated prediction*, *service management strategy design and evaluation*, and *behavior-based autonomy-oriented modeling*, to address practical healthcare service management problems. This chapter presents an intelligent healthcare decision support (iHDS) system that implements the four methods to develop, analyze, investigate, support, and provide advice for healthcare-related decisions. The iHDS system provides the architecture and components for user interactions, data collection and processing, data-driven inferences and simulations, and decision analytics and support to generate solutions for various healthcare analytics and decision-making problems. This chapter also describes two cases to illustrate how the iHDS system works to address practical healthcare analytics problems. One case illustrates how the components and methods work to generate adaptive solutions for allocating time blocks in operating rooms (ORs), while the other addresses the need for adaptive decision support in regional healthcare resource allocation that has the advantage of reducing healthcare performance disparities.

8.1 Introduction

Healthcare decision analytics and support serve as the most crucial functions for healthcare-service-providing organizations, practitioners, researchers, decision makers, patients, general users, and other relevant stakeholders. To demonstrate how the data-driven complex systems modeling approach (D^2CSM) can be implemented to address practical decision analytics and support problems in this chapter, we provide a comprehensive design of our iHDS system. This system (1) helps users extract and infer, integrate, fuse, and interpret healthcare-related information; (2) provides various functions and techniques to scientifically develop, analyze,

© Springer Nature Switzerland AG 2019
L. Tao, J. Liu, *Healthcare Service Management*, Health Information Science,
https://doi.org/10.1007/978-3-030-15385-4_8

and evaluate healthcare related decisions for services and operations, such as OR time block assignments (discussed in Chap. 6), that involve many dynamically-interacting endogenous and exogenous impact factors (discussed in Chaps. 4 and 5) in multiple temporal or spatial scales (discussed in Chap. 7); and (3) produces evidence-based recommendations and analytics support for users.

Potential users of the iHDS system include healthcare administrators at a regional level and an individual health service level, healthcare-service-providing organizations, such as hospitals and labs, healthcare workers, such as doctors and nurses, stakeholders, such as secondary service providers and patients (here, patients should be understood in a broad sense, and include all the potential healthcare service users). For instance, regional (e.g., a country, a province, a city, or a district) healthcare administrators can be supported by the iHDS system when they plan and allocate healthcare resources and propose strategies and procedures for public healthcare infrastructure and services. Hospital and other healthcare service administrators can use the iHDS system as an aid when they analyze, evaluate, and predict the outcomes and efficacy of their strategies and operations, e.g., in scheduling physical and human resources and smoothing out the logistic processes among different units. Healthcare-service-providing organizations and healthcare workers, such as doctors, may be assisted by the iHDS system to help them make their clinical decisions about treating patients based on evidence derived from different sources, such as historical patient clinical data and academic/medical research findings. Patients can benefit in their own health related decisions (e.g., daily care, doctor, or treatment selections), as the iHDS system offers evidence-based information and decision suggestions with respect to their own specific profiles.

Users can access the iHDS system and present their analytics and decision problems in any centralized, distributed, and pervasive manner. The objective(s), problem types, issues, sub-questions, criteria, requirements (e.g., indicators and measurements), and corresponding decision or control variables and constraints for the decision analytics problem will be automatically extracted or inferred from the users' problem sketches or descriptions. The iHDS system extracts or infers the contextual information for the users and analytics problem at hand, such as the users' profiles and the scope of the analytics problem (e.g., the decision analytics and supports for a region or for a hospital). The system has the ability to record and recall encountered users and to automatically identify or infer the types of subsequent users with their profiles and relate their needs (i.e., required decision analytics and support problems) together, to intelligently and automatically infer and recommend the decision analytics problems for subsequent users.

Five major categories of data sources will be utilized by the iHDS system to achieve the objectives of different healthcare analytics and decision problems. The first major category of data sources corresponds to the existing healthcare service operations, including patient profiles and clinical information from actual healthcare systems, as well as investment, policies, and management information, both at a regional level and an individual healthcare service level. The second category of data sources relates to ubiquitous patient data, including personal information (e.g., personal profiles and daily activities), patient health information routinely collected from ubiquitous devices (e.g., smart phones), and clinical and patient information distributed in health related physical and online communities (e.g., forums). The third category of data sources comes from the healthcare-related secondary service providers, such as community health service centers, rehabilitation centers, insurance companies, pharmacy companies, and medical apparatus and instruments companies. The fourth data source relates to the exogenous factors, dynamic or static, which affect the inputs of actual healthcare service systems (e.g., geodemographic-, environmental-, and socioeconomic-related factors, as well as human behavior), and serve as the essential contexts for healthcare-related decisions. Finally, academic/medical research databases will be incorporated into the iHDS system with prior academic/medical research findings to be utilized for healthcare evidential inferences, hypothesis generations, and model constructions, as well as to discover explicit and implicit relationships among impact factors and decision parameters and variables, e.g., drug-drug interactions in drug development.

The iHDS system is able to identify, infer, and support the analytics and decision-making tasks at different service scales, depending on users' decision-making needs and requirements. The analytics techniques, which will be used either individually or in an integrated manner depending on the specific tasks at hand, include statistical analysis tools (e.g., regression, ANOVA, and SEM), intelligent analysis tools (e.g., artificial intelligence, machine learning, and data mining techniques), and intelligent complex-healthcare-systems modeling and strategic analysis tools (e.g., AOC-based modeling and queueing modeling), optimization and intelligent computation tools (e.g., mathematical programming), numerical or agent-based simulation tools, and visualization tools. This intelligently configured and integrated processing capability allows for producing solutions to practical healthcare decision analytics problems that involve complex-systems behavior and a large number of intrinsic or extrinsic interactive impact factors.

8.2 An Overview of the iHDS System

Figure 8.1 schematically illustrates the key modules for the iHDS system, i.e., the Intelligent User Interface, Healthcare Decision Analytics and Support System (HDASS) module, and Information Management System (IMS) module, as well as its interactions with users and healthcare-related data.

The Intelligent User Interface is capable of (1) permitting users to access the iHDS system in any centralized, distributed, or pervasive manner and to input their sketches or descriptions of analytics and decision problems, as well as to optionally modify the solution repository, settings, and configurations; (2) extracting or inferring the contextual information for users and analytics problems at hand; (3) extracting, inferring, or refining objective(s), problem types, issues, sub-questions, criteria, requirements (e.g., indicators and measurements), and the corresponding decisions or constraints for the decision analytics problems; (4) intelligently inferring and recommending the decision analytics problems for subsequent

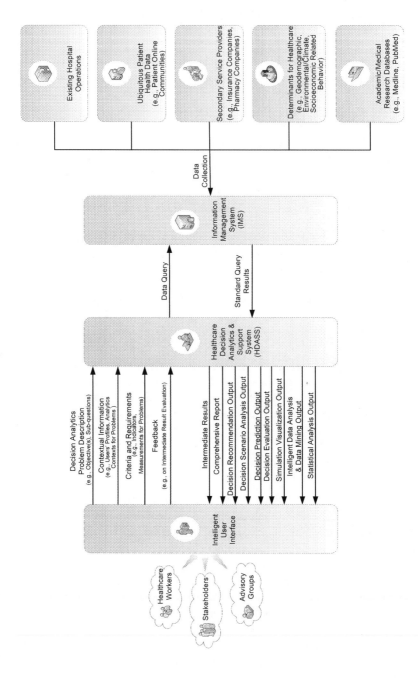

Fig. 8.1 Key modules in the intelligent healthcare decision support system

users; and (5) extracting or inferring feedback from users (e.g., on the intermediate result evaluations) during the analytics process.

The IMS module collects, preprocesses, and maintains the data collected from Existing Hospital Operations (e.g., databases of electronic health records (EHR), electronic medical records (EMR), the hospital information system (HIS), and the management information system (MIS)), Ubiquitous Patient Health Data Sources (e.g., patient online communities), Secondary Service Providers (e.g., insurance companies and pharmacy companies), Determinants for Healthcare (e.g., geodemographic, environmental, climate, socioeconomic related behavior), and Academic/ Medical Research Databases (e.g., Medline and PubMed). It contains information buses for handling database inputs and communications between the HDASS and IMS in any centralized, distributed, or pervasive manner.

The most important component in the iHDS system is HDASS. HDASS receives the input information from users through either an integrated or a distributed user-HDASS interface. With an analytics engine, HDASS extracts and infers the desired type of problems (e.g., whether they are optimization problems or statistical analysis problems) and the desired issues to be addressed for users (e.g., which candidate techniques should be chosen and how the selected techniques are individually, sequentially, iteratively, or integrally used) from the input information. HDASS then determines, accesses, retrieves, organizes, and preprocesses the required data for analytics. After that, HDASS generates analytics solutions, performs the analytics tasks based on the empirical and secondary data stored, maintained, and integrated in the information management system (IMS), and intelligently fine-tunes the solutions according to users' criteria, requirements, and feedback on the intermediate results during the analytics, investigation, and simulation processes. At the end of the analytics process, HDASS returns the analytics results in the form of comprehensive textual or graphical reports, with outputs of recommendations, scenario analyses, predictions, evaluations, visualizations, intelligent data analysis, data mining, and statistical analysis. Furthermore, it retains the resulting healthcare decision analytics solutions (i.e., in terms of the generalized flows of problem-solving with respect to the computational types, issues, and sub-questions of the decision analytics problems, instead of the exact instances of the problems) in its solution repository, such that the accumulatively aggregated solutions in the repository can be stored, inter-connected, updated, and utilized for tackling similar or more complex types, issues, and sub-questions of future problems.

The analytics engine in HDASS implements and intelligently deploys three main groups of analytics methods. The first and most important group of methods is for strategic analysis. Exemplified methods in this group include techniques for algorithmic or mechanism design, exact or approximate queueing modeling, discrete event simulation, optimization (e.g., mathematical programming), and AOC-based modeling. This group of methods, integrated with the following two groups if needed, is especially useful in solving complex decision analytics problems. The second group of analytics methods consists of intelligent data analysis methods, such as artificial intelligence techniques, machine learning techniques, data mining techniques, and pattern recognition techniques. The third group of analytics methods encompasses data-driven statistical analysis methods, such as regression, ANOVA, structural equation modeling, and factor analysis.

Depending on different decision analytics and support problems, the three groups of analytics methods will be utilized either individually, sequentially, iteratively, or in any integrated manner, depending on the specific tasks at hand. For instance, in some cases, the results of data-driven analysis will be used to support the further intelligent data analysis and the strategic analysis tasks; the intelligent data analysis results will also feed the strategic analysis methods. In other cases, the three groups of analytics methods, as well as their underlying possessed techniques, will be integrally utilized, e.g., the simulation, evaluation, and prediction results obtained from the strategic analysis will be further investigated by employing data-driven analysis or intelligent data analysis.

8.3   Key Components of the iHDS System

The operations of the Intelligent User Interface and the HDASS and IMS modules are executed by their components, as shown in the drawing in Fig. 8.2. Users access the iHDS system aided by the User Accessing component within the Intelligent User Interface module. Functions of the Collecting Decision Analytics Problem Description component permit users to present their decision analytics problems and then automatically extract, infer, and refine the objective(s), problem types, issues, sub-questions, criteria, requirements (e.g., indicators and measurements), and corresponding decision or control variables and constraints for the decision analytics problem. The User Profiling component extracts or infers the contextual information for users and the analytics problem, such as the users' profiles and analytics scale of the problem (e.g., decision analytics and supports for a region or for a hospital) during the user-system interaction process. With the functions provided by the component of Inferring and Recommending User's Needs in Decision Analytics, the Intelligent User Interface is able to record and recall the encountered users and identify and infer the types of subsequent users with their profiles and relate their needs (i.e., the required decision analytics and support problems) together, so as to intelligently infer and recommend the decision analytics problems for subsequent users. The Intelligent User Interface module runs consistently during the analytics processes to gather and incorporate user-initiated feedback (e.g., on the intermediate result evaluation), and intelligently infer feedback on behalf of users by Gathering User-Initiated Feedback or Intelligently Inferring Feedback on the Intermediate Results.

Data stored, maintained, and integrated in the IMS module are collected from five major data sources related to healthcare. The first typical data sources included in the present iHDS system are the existing hospital operations databases, such as electronic health records databases (EHR), electronic medical records (EMR) databases, hospital information system (HIS) databases, and management information system (MIS) databases. Ubiquitous patient health data form the second

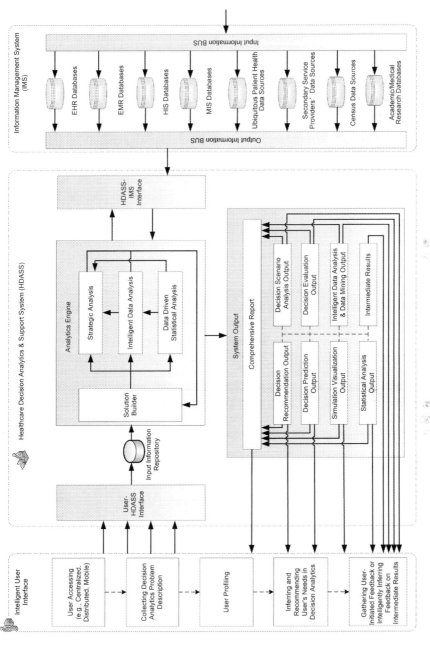

Fig. 8.2 Key components of the Intelligent User Interface module, HDASS module, IMS module, and the relevant interactions

major data source. Ubiquitous patient health data include personal information (e.g., personal profiles and daily activities) and patient health information routinely collected from ubiquitous devices (e.g., smart phones), and clinical and patient information (e.g., experiences of treatments and medication) distributed in health-related physical and online communities (e.g., forums). IMS also contains data from secondary service providers related to healthcare, such as community health service centers, rehabilitation centers, insurance companies, pharmacy companies, and medical apparatus and instruments companies. Since the demand for healthcare services is constantly affected by certain exogenous factors to the healthcare system, primary and secondary data on the determinants for healthcare, such as demographic (usually represented by census data), environmental, climate, and socioeconomic factors and human behavior, are gathered, stored, and tracked in IMS. The fifth and final data source integrated in the iHDS system encompasses medical research and other relevant databases, such as Medline and PubMed, which feed the HDASS with prior academic research findings. These data sources are utilized for healthcare evidential inferences, hypothesis generation, and model construction, as well as for discovering explicit and implicit relationships among the impact factors and decision parameters and variables, e.g., drug-drug interactions in drug development. In IMS, those data sources are collected, cleaned, and integrated through an input information bus. The preprocessed data in IMS then support the decision analytics and tasks in HDASS by a standard query through an output information bus. The iHDS system described herein is susceptible to variations and modifications other than those specifically described.

The HDASS module offers methods for recognizing and inferring decision analytics problems, building and fine-tuning solutions, supporting techniques, and automatically generating various kinds of outputs (e.g., decision recommendation output and statistical analytics output) for users. With a User-HDASS Interface, the output of the Intelligent User Interface component (i.e., the Decision Analytics Problem Description, Contextual Information, Criteria and Requirements, and Feedback) will be temporarily stored in the Input Information Repository, from which the Solution Builder within the Analytics Engine will then be invoked to (1) recognize and infer problems (e.g., types, issues, and sub-questions) to be addressed, select suitable solutions and intelligently integrate the suitable techniques (i.e., generate a solution for an analytics task); (2) determine the necessary data sources for analytics and access, retrieve, organize, and preprocess the needed data queried by the HDASS-IMS Interface from IMS to parameterize and support various analytics and decision-making tasks; (3) operate the components of the Strategic Analysis, Intelligent Data Analysis, and Data-Driven Statistical Analysis individually or in an integrated manner upon receiving the treated data; (4) intelligently fine-tune the solution, as well as the parameter settings in the solution, according to the users' criteria and requirements as well as the extracted or inferred contextual information; (5) return the intermediate and final analytics results automatically generated by the Comprehensive Report, Decision Recommendation Output, Decision Scenario Analysis Output, Decision Prediction Output, Decision Evaluation Output, Simulation Visualization Output, Intelligent Data Analysis and Data Mining Output,

Statistical Analysis Output, and Intermediate Results; and (6) retain the resulting healthcare decision analytics solutions (i.e., in terms of the generalized flows of problem-solving with respect to the computational types, issues, and sub-questions of the decision analytics problems, instead of the exact instances of the problems) in its solution repository. The accumulatively aggregated solutions in the repository then can be stored, inter-connected, updated, and utilized for managing similar or more complex types, issues, and sub-questions of future problems.

The functions and examples of the integrated techniques provided by the Analytics Engine of the HDASS module are presented in the drawing shown in Fig. 8.3. The Identifying Problem Types sub-module within the Solution Builder, supported by the functions of Semantic Analysis (e.g., XML-based, HL 7 Standards-based) and Problem Classification and Matching, will help to infer the type and the scope of the analytics problems (e.g., optimization problems or statistical analysis problems or a combination of both problem types) and issues or sub-questions to be addressed by the Input Information Repository.

With respect to the identified problem types, scope, issues, and sub-questions, the Determining Solution sub-module will choose suitable existing solutions and intelligently extend, revise, customize, or integrate the suitable techniques (i.e., generate a solution for an analytics task) to build new solutions by calling the Retrieving Existing Solutions, Meta-Knowledge About the Relationship Between Problems and Solutions, and Required Analytics Techniques Extension/Customization/Revise/Integration. The techniques categorized in the Strategic Analysis, Intelligent Data Analysis, and Data-Driven Statistical Analysis sub-modules will be used individually, sequentially, or in an integrated manner for solving the decision analytics problems.

During the analytics process, the Determining Solution sub-module will monitor and evaluate the automatically built solution based on the users' criteria, requirements, and feedback on the intermediate results, so as to automatically and intelligently improve the solution by calling the Fine-Tuning Solution. The updated or newly-built solutions will be incrementally stored and maintained in the Maintaining Solution sub-module by calling the Updating Personalized Solution Information and Updating Technique Repositories of Strategic Analysis/Intelligent Data Analysis/Data-Driven Statistical Analysis sub-modules. This function of the iHDS system allows for the solutions to be accumulatively aggregated for future reuse.

The Solution Builder component also determines the needed data sources for analytics by Determining Required Data Sources within Acquiring Required Data, and prepares the needed data by calling Required Data Accessing, Retrieving, Organizing, and Preprocessing to support various data analytics and data-driven modeling steps.

Before executing the techniques already chosen and extended, customized, revised, and integrated in the solution, the Configuring Solution sub-module of the Solution Builder will initialize and parameterize the techniques with the related variables by calling Initializing and Parameterizing Techniques in Solution. During the analytics process, the Configuring Solution sub-module will automatically and

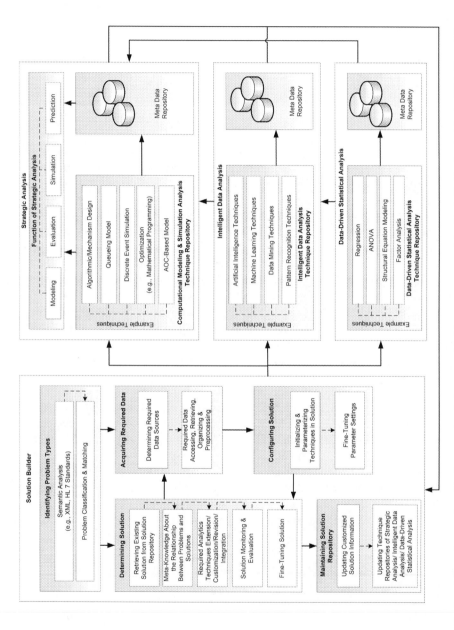

Fig. 8.3 The functions and examples of the integrated techniques provided by a component of the Analytics Engine inside the HDASS module

intelligently fine-tune the parameter settings in the solution according to users' criteria and requirements, contextual information, intermediate analytics results, and users' feedback by calling Fine-Tuning Parameter Settings.

After the intelligent selection and composition of the decision analytics and support techniques in providing the solution(s) via Solution Builder, the Analytics Engine will execute the techniques categorized as Strategic Analysis, Intelligent Data Analysis, and Data-Driven Statistical Analysis. In the Strategic Analysis sub-module, the functions include Modeling, Evaluation, Simulation, and Predication for selected strategies, where techniques from Computational Modeling and Simulation Analysis Technique Repository, as exemplified by the Algorithmic/Mechanism Design, Queueing Model, Discrete Event Simulation, Optimization (such as mathematical programming), and AOC-Based Model, will be used. The Strategic Analysis phase will be carried out separately, or based on the results from the Intelligent Data Analysis and the Data-Driven Statistical Analysis phases and vice versa (i.e., providing results to Intelligent Data Analysis and Data-Driven Statistical Analysis). In Intelligent Data Analysis, the data analysis functions will be achieved by utilizing techniques in Intelligent Data Analysis Technique Repository, as exemplified by Artificial Intelligence Techniques, Machine Learning Techniques, Data Mining Techniques, and Pattern Recognition Techniques. The Intelligent Data Analysis phase will also be executed based on the result from the Data-Driven Statistical Analysis phase (and vice versa), in which techniques from Data-Driven Statistical Analysis Technique Repository, as exemplified by Regression, ANOVA, Structural Equation Modeling, and Factor Analysis, will be used.

8.4   Case 1: Adaptive OR Time Block Allocation

The drawing in Fig. 8.4 presents the key modules for the first case (i.e., the Intelligent User Interface, the HDASS module, and the IMS module), and their interactions with the users (i.e., as healthcare workers) and healthcare-related data collected from Existing Hospital Operations. The drawing in Fig. 8.5 shows the sub-modules within the Analytics Engine in the first case, which includes the processes and methods in the Solution Builder and Strategic Analysis modules, respectively.

After users access the iHDS system via the User Accessing component of the Intelligent User Interface in any centralized, distributed or pervasive manner, the Collecting Decision Analytics Problem Description component within the Intelligent User Interface module will collect the general description of the problem (i.e., how can OR time blocks be adaptively allocated to maintain a stable OR performance in the face of dynamically-changing and non-deterministic patient arrivals?). The User Profiling component of the Intelligent User Interface module extracts and infers the contextual information for the user and the analytics problem, such as whether the user type is a hospital administrator or the work place and analytics context are the cardiac surgery ORs in the Hamilton Health Science Centre.

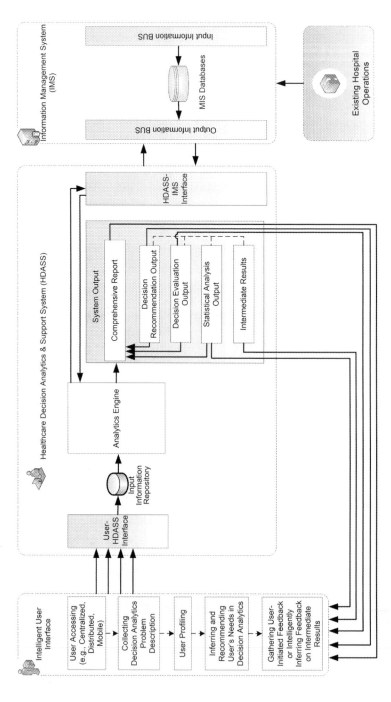

Fig. 8.4 The components, functions, and employed techniques in the first case that uses the iHDS system to design adaptive strategies for OR time block allocation

Fig. 8.5 The employed techniques and specific processes within the Analytics Engine module in the first case for designing adaptive strategies for the OR time block allocation

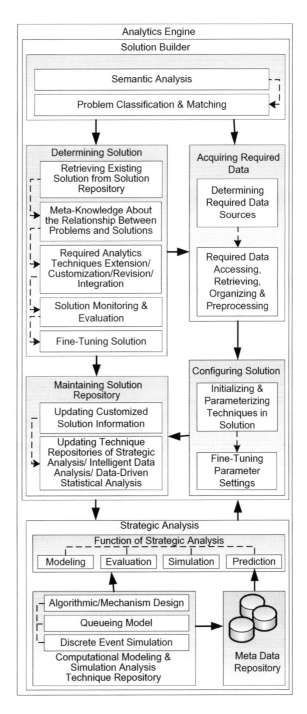

The objective(s), problem types, issues, sub-questions, criteria, requirements (e.g., indicators and measurements), and corresponding decision variables and constraints for the decision analytics problem will be extracted, inferred, and refined from the users' problem sketches or descriptions. For instance, the objective should be to provide an adaptive method for OR time block allocation. For instance, the inferred sub-questions may include: (1) how to characterize dynamically-changing and non-deterministic patient arrivals, (2) how to characterize the operations of ORs, and (3) what mechanism helps to adaptively allocate OR time blocks for unpredictable patients with different urgent levels. The criteria and requirements include the trade-off between the number of bumped non-urgent surgeries and unused urgent time blocks, the average wait times for measuring the performance of ORs, and the dynamics of wait times with or without the produced adaptive OR time block allocation method.

Upon the inputs from the Decision Analytics Problem Description (e.g., objective(s), problem types, issues, and sub-questions), Contextual Information (e.g., users' profiles and analytics context for problems), and Criteria and Requirements components from the Intelligent User Interface, the Solution Builder of the HDASS module identifies and infers the problem types based on the functions provided by Semantic Analysis and Problem Classification and Matching sub-modules within the Solution Builder. According to the problem sketch from the user and the inferred objective, problem type, issues, sub-questions, contextual information, criteria, requirements (e.g., indicators and measurements), and corresponding decision variables and constraints, the problem will be solved by integrating mechanism design-based optimization along with simulation-based evaluation, and the ORs' wait time dynamics demonstration.

To build a solution to achieve the analytics objective and to answer the sub-questions, the Retrieving Existing Solution from Solution Repository and Meta-Knowledge About the Relationship Between Problems and Solutions sub-modules within the Determine Solution component automatically find that the Queueing Model and Discrete Event Simulation from the Computational Modeling and Simulation Analysis Technique Repository within the Strategic Analysis component are useful approaches for modeling and simulating the operations of ORs' existing solutions. The Solution Builder then automatically and intelligently builds a solution that sequentially utilizes Algorithmic/Mechanism Design to produce an adaptive OR time block allocation strategy, Queueing Model to model the operations of ORs, and Discrete Event Simulation to simulate the proposed queueing model with an adaptive OR time block allocation strategy to evaluate (in terms of the trade-off between the number of bumped non-urgent surgeries and unused urgent time blocks for the ORs' time block allocation and the average wait times for measuring the performance of ORs) and fine-tune the produced adaptive OR time block allocation method through the functions of Fine-Tuning Solution.

The Acquiring Required Data sub-module of the Solution Builder determines and accesses the necessary data sources for developing, parameterizing, analyzing, and evaluating the adaptive OR time block allocation method aided by the functions of Determining Required Data Sources and Required Data Accessing, Retrieving, Organizing and Preprocessing.

IMS collects and stores the necessary data for parameterizing, simulating, and evaluating the method of adaptive OR time block allocation for the existing operations at the Hamilton Health Sciences Centre (HHSC) in Centralized/Distributed/Pervasive MIS Databases. The HHSC contains six specialized surgeons and two operating rooms, and provides 1400 cardiac surgeries annually. Table 6.1 is an example that shows a summary of the HHSC cardiac surgery data.

Aided by the functions of Initializing and Parameterizing Techniques in Solution of Configuring Solution within the Analytics Engine, this case utilizes the data to initialize the parameter settings of the adaptive OR time block allocation method, the corresponding queueing model, and the subsequent discrete event simulations.

To achieve the objective of adaptive OR time block allocation, Algorithmic/Mechanism Design in the Analytics Engine within HDASS produces an adaptive OR time block allocation scheduler based on a feedback mechanism (refer to Fig. 6.2). The main idea of this case is to adjust time blocks for urgent surgeries periodically based on the feedback information corresponding to the arrivals of different priority groups and the effectiveness of ORs. Specifically, this adaptive method utilizes an adjusted window mechanism, which is shown in Fig. 6.3.

To present the performance of the disclosed adaptive method, this case has specifically built a queueing model (refer to Fig. 6.4) based on the empirical data on cardiac surgery operating rooms in HHSC. The Discrete Event Simulation is utilized to simulate the queueing model. The simulations are carried out based on the HHSC statistical data. To compare the performance, the exemplified system carries out the simulations under the same conditions after a single run. It can also perform multiple simulation runs.

In the first case, System Output within HDASS includes Decision Evaluation Output for the queueing model and the adaptive OR time block allocation method by simulations, Decision Recommendation Output for result findings, and Comprehensive Report comprising the simulation results, sensitivity analysis for key parameters (e.g., the adjustment step sizes and the thresholds) of the adaptive OR scheduling strategy, Decision Evaluation Output and Decision Recommendation Output. Figure 6.5 shows the Decision Evaluation Output for evaluating the effectiveness of the adaptive OR time block allocation method in terms of the queue length. Figures 6.6 and 6.7 show another two outputs as the exemplified Decision Evaluation Output. Figure 6.6 shows that the adaptive method can reduce the number of bumped non-urgent surgeries. Figure 6.7 shows the changes in the OR time blocks for urgent surgeries with the adaptive strategy over time.

The Decision Recommendation Output in the first case contains the following recommendations: (1) the generated adaptive OR time block allocation method is able to more efficiently regulate the OR time block reservation in accordance with the changing pattern of patient arrivals; (2) the hospital OR scheduler employing the generated adaptive method can maintain a better trade-off between the number of bumped non-urgent surgeries and the number of unused urgent OR time blocks;

and (3) frequently adjusting the OR time block allocation (i.e., once per week or per month) can improve the ORs' effectiveness. The Comprehensive Report comprising the above-mentioned evaluation outputs and decision recommendation outputs is also generated for users.

8.5   Case 2: Adaptive Regional Healthcare Resource Allocation

Healthcare resource allocation is an important problem for regional healthcare administrators. Prior research [130] has advocated allocating resources according to the occurrence and harmfulness of diseases in the population, for instance, as assessed by the population-needs-based funding formula based on neighborhood geodemographic factors (e.g., population size, age profile, geographic accessibility to services, and educational profile). However, examining traditional estimation methods for service needs, such as those introduced in prior research [146], shows there are substantial differences between the estimated and real needs in some regions. A possible explanation for the biased estimation is that the needs estimation method is simply a linear combination of the considered factors that does not take into consideration how these factors interact with each another as well as how patients' behavior relates to healthcare.

Imagine that you are a regional healthcare administrator in Ontario. You find that the current resource allocation method for cardiac surgery services is static and results in a gap between the estimated and real needs in LHINs. Therefore, you would like to make a reasonable and evidence-based decision on regional resource allocation for cardiac surgery to shorten the regional average wait times and reduce wait time disparities. You seek help from the iHDS system and design your decision analytics and support problem as follows:

"How can I adaptively allocate cardiac surgery resources in Ontario to shorten the provincial average wait time and reduce wait time disparities in the face of dynamically-changing and non-deterministic patient arrivals?"

After receiving your request and the general problem description, the iHDS system intelligently identifies and infers the objective(s), problem types, issues, sub-questions, contextual information, criteria, requirements (e.g., indicators and measurements), and corresponding decision variables and constraints, builds a solution, employs or customizes the identified techniques for decision analysis, and returns an adaptive regional resource allocation method, statistical and strategic analysis outputs, decision evaluation, and recommendation outputs. In what follows, we will show the operational process, methods and components of the present iHDS system involved in the second case to: (1) analyze the relationships between neighborhood geodemographic factors and cardiac surgery characteristics (e.g., the number of patient arrivals) pertaining to the hospitals; (2) model patient arrival behavior and cardiac surgery service operations in the hospitals to investigate the temporal-spatial patterns of service utilizations and complex emergent behavior (i.e., behavior of a complex healthcare system, such as reneging behavior in hospital selection) of the exemplified cardiac surgery service through simulation; and (3) automatically generate an adaptive method for allocating regional cardiac surgery resources based on simulations.

The drawing in Fig. 8.6 presents the key modules involved in the second test case of the iHDS system, i.e., the Intelligent User Interface, the HDASS, and the IMS modules, and its interactions (e.g., through the intermediate results and user's feedback on them) with the user (e.g., you, as a healthcare worker) via the Intelligent User Interface and necessary healthcare-related data about Existing Hospital Operations, Determinants for Healthcare (e.g., demographic and socioeconomic related behavior), and Academic/Medical Research Databases.

The drawing in Fig. 8.7 shows the sub-modules within the Analytics Engine for the second case, which includes the processes and methods in the Solution Builder, Strategic Analysis, and Data-Driven Statistical Analysis modules, respectively.

After you access the iHDS system via the User Accessing component of the Intelligent User Interface in any centralized, distributed, or pervasive manner, the Collecting Decision Analytics Problem Description component of the Intelligent User Interface will gather the general description of the problem (i.e., How can I adaptively allocate cardiac surgery resources in Ontario to shorten the province's average wait times and reduce wait time disparities in the face of dynamically-changing and non-deterministic patient arrivals?).

The User Profiling component of the Intelligent User Interface module extracts and infers the contextual information for the user (i.e., you, in this case) and the analytics problem, such as the user type is a provincial healthcare service administrator and the analytics context is the cardiac surgery services in Ontario. The objective(s), problem types, issues, sub-questions, criteria, requirements (e.g., indicators and measurements), and corresponding decision variables and constraints for the decision analytics problem will be automatically extracted, inferred, and refined from the user's problem and the extracted or inferred contextual information. For instance, the objective is to provide an adaptive method for regional healthcare resource allocation in order to shorten the regional average wait times and reduce regional wait time disparities. Sub-questions will involve: (1) what and how geodemographic factors affect the cardiac surgery service characteristics (e.g., the number of patient arrivals and wait times), (2) how to model patient service utilization behavior, so as to characterize dynamically-changing and non-deterministic patient arrivals to investigate the temporal-spatial patterns of cardiac surgery service utilizations, and even to capture the emergent behavior (e.g., reneging behavior in hospital selection) of the exemplified complex healthcare system, (3) how to characterize the operations of cardiac surgery services, and (4) what mechanism helps to adaptively allocate the cardiac surgery resources with respect to the regional heterogeneity in terms of geodemographic factors and the patient heterogeneity in terms of health service utilization behavior. Examples of the criteria and requirements include the measurement of regional wait time disparities,

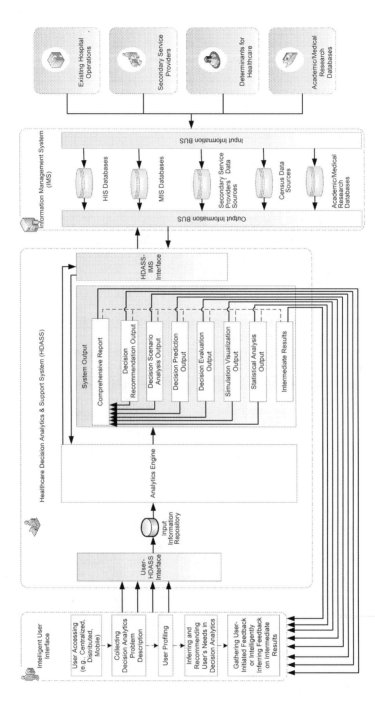

Fig. 8.6 The components, functions, and employed techniques in the second test case of utilizing the iHDS system to adaptively allocate regional healthcare resources

Fig. 8.7 The sub-modules
with specific processes and
employed techniques within
the Analytics Engine module
in the second case of utilizing
the iHDS system

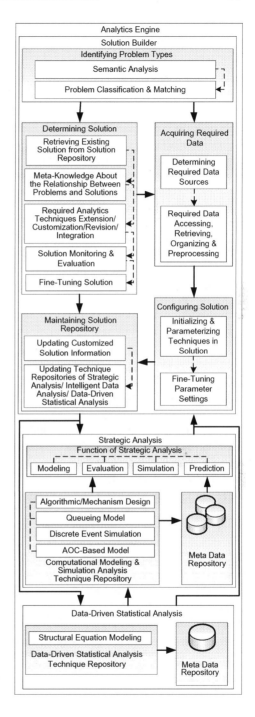

the temporal-spatial patterns, and the dynamically-changing process of regional patient arrivals and wait times for cardiac surgery services.

Upon the input from the Intelligent User Interface module about the decision analytical problem description (e.g., objective(s) and sub-questions), the contextual information (e.g., users' profiles and analytics context for problems), and the criteria and requirements components, the HDASS Solution Builder identifies the problem types based on the functions provided by the embedded Semantic Analysis and Problem Classification and Matching sub-modules. According to the problem defined by the user and the inferred objective, problem type, issues, sub-questions, contextual information, criteria, requirements (e.g., indicators and measurements), and corresponding decision variables and constraints, the problem will be solved by integrating the statistical analysis, mechanism design, modeling and simulation, and optimization.

To build a solution to achieve the analytics objective(s) and answer the sub-questions, the Retrieving Existing Solution from Solution Repository and Meta-Knowledge About the Relationship Between Problems and Solutions within the Determine Solution automatically infers that: (1) SEM is suitable for modeling and analyzing the complex and hierarchical relationships between geodemographic factors and cardiac surgery service characteristics in that it is efficient in constructing latent variables (i.e., variables that cannot be measured directly) and testing complex relationships among the observed and latent variables, as explained by Hair et al. [48]; (2) the AOC-Based Model is in favor of modeling the cardiac surgery system with respect to patient service utilization behavior; (3) the Queueing Model and Discrete Event Simulation modules from the Computational Modeling and Simulation Analysis Technique Repository within the Strategic Analysis sub-modules are useful approaches to modeling and simulating the operations of ORs; and (4) Simulation-Based Optimization is beneficial to generate an adaptive resource allocation method through simulation independently or based on the Algorithmic/Mechanism Design.

The Solution Builder then automatically and intelligently builds a solution that integrally utilizes Structural Equation Modeling, AOC-Based Model, Queueing Model, Discrete Event Simulation, Algorithmi/Mechanism Design, and Simulation-Based Optimization to achieve the objective(s) of the user and answer the closely-interrelated sub-questions. Specifically, the AOC-based modeling of the cardiac surgery system with respect to patient service utilization behavior (i.e., arrival behavior) will refer to the SEM results. The AOC-based cardiac surgery model comprises a specific queueing model for service operations. Both AOC-based multi-agent simulations and discrete event simulations will together support the implementation of Simulation-Based Optimization.

Accordingly, the Acquiring Required Data component of the Solution Builder determines and accesses the necessary data sources for this analytics problem aided by the functions of the Determining Required Data Sources and Required Data Accessing, Retrieving, Organizing and Preprocessing. The data sources involved in this analytics problem contain Existing Hospital Operations (about the characteristics of cardiac surgery services), Secondary Service Provider (e.g., about the referral for cardiac surgery from family doctors), and Determinants for Healthcare (e.g., the geodemographic profiles for a region).

IMS has collected, stored, and maintained the necessary data for developing, parameterizing, analyzing, modeling, simulating, and evaluating of the adaptive resource allocation problem. The HIS and MIS databases contain data representing cardiac surgery characteristics (i.e., arrival, capacity, supply, and wait time) in Ontario, Canada, in the years between 2004 and 2007. The databases of Census Data Sources have stored neighborhood geodemographic data gathered from the 2006 Canadian Census with respect to the population size, age profile, and educational profile. In this illustration, 47 major cities/towns in Ontario with populations of more than 40,000 (this population cut-off point was determined so that the cities/towns included in the sample represented approximately 90.72% of Ontario's population) were selected to derive the geodemographic profiles for 14 LHINs. In addition, the Secondary Service Providers' databases collected and stored the driving time from each sampled city or town to the nearest hospital that provides cardiac surgery services to measure service accessibility. In this illustration, the driving times were estimated based on the "Get Directions" function in Google Maps.

For the solution, the iHDS system in the second case first automatically (1) builds hypotheses based on the previous studies stored and maintained in Centralized/Distributed/Pervasive Academic/Medical Research Databases, in which data were gathered from Academic/Medical Research Databases (e.g., Medline and PubMed), and (2) utilizes the SEM method to capture the relationships between geodemographic factors and patient arrivals for cardiac surgery services based on the data queried from the HIS Databases, MIS Databases, and Secondary Service Providers' Data Sources.

According to the determined solution, the iHDS system in the second case automatically and intelligently models the cardiac surgery system considering patient arrival behavior based on the findings of the SEM test and AOC-based modeling to identify and evaluate the dynamics of patient arrivals and wait times and capture the complex emergent behavior of the healthcare system. In the AOC-Based Cardiac Surgery System Model, the behavior of three types of autonomous behavior-based entities, i.e., patient, GP, and hospital, their behavioral interactions, as well as the environment actively carrying out information exchanges, are automatically and computationally modeled.

As suggested by the preceding SEM-based Statistical Analysis Output and prior studies [29], the major factors that should be considered in modeling autonomous patients'/GPs' hospital selection behavior include the quantities of healthcare physical (e.g., the number of operating rooms) and human resources (e.g., the number of physicians), the geographic distance from home to hospitals, and the waiting time for receiving the requested healthcare services. As in the actual cardiac surgery system, patients almost follow GPs' referral suggestions. Therefore, the iHDS system sets that autonomous patient entities always select the hospital that is recommended by their GPs.

The autonomous hospital selection behavior of a GP is automatically and computationally modeled based on the following decision process. When GP entities choose a hospital, they will first calculate the utility (representing the degree of satisfaction on a hospital in terms of the travel distance, service quality assurance, and wait times for receiving services) for each hospital based on released information and their experience on historical referrals in terms of wait times. The hospital that has the highest expected utility will be recommended.

The autonomous behavior of hospital entities is automatically and computationally modeled based on queueing processes. Thus, in the second case, the Queueing Model proposed a general Multi-Priority, Multi-Server, Non-Preemptive Queueing Model for a hospital.

Based on the AOC-based cardiac surgery system model described earlier, discrete-event simulations were carried out to validate the model and to examine the temporal-spatial service utilization patterns, the dynamics of patient arrivals and healthcare service performance in terms of the throughput, wait times, and queue length, and the emergent behavior of the complex healthcare system in different scenarios. In addition, adaptive methods and strategies for healthcare resource allocation were generated, evaluated, and recommended by means of AOC-based (i.e., AOC-by-self-discovery) modeling and simulation.

The second case provides decision analytics and support in the form of the textual or graphical Comprehensive Report, Decision Recommendation Output, Decision Scenario Analysis Output, Decision Prediction Output, Decision Evaluation Output, Simulation Visualization Output, and Statistical Analysis Output. In particular, the generated SEM testing results and suggestions for healthcare resource allocation are formatted and reported by the Statistical Analysis Output and Decision Recommendation Output in the module of System Output within HDASS. In Decision Recommendation Output, the generated findings of the SEM testing results suggest that: (1) regional wait time disparities in cardiac surgery services are associated with differences in geodemographic profiles, such as service accessibility and education; (2) the allocation of resources for a particular healthcare service in one area should consider the geographic distribution of the same service in neighboring areas; and (3) an increase in physician resources and the more efficient use of existing surgical facilities may contribute to a reduction in cardiac surgery wait time.

Built on the above results, the simulation results of the AOC-based cardiac surgery system modeling and the following strategic analysis on adaptive healthcare resource allocation are generated, formatted, and reported in the forms of the textual or graphical Comprehensive Report, Decision Recommendation Output, Decision Scenario Analysis Output, Decision Prediction Output, Decision Evaluation Output, and Simulation Visualization Output. After being parameterized by the actual geodemographic and hospital characteristics data, the AOC-based cardiac surgery system model is validated by autonomous behavior-based simulations. The temporal-spatial hospital service utilization patterns and the dynamics of patient arrivals and hospital performance are generated and observed. Then, based on the validated AOC-based cardiac surgery system model, simulations are run in different scenarios (e.g., a sharp increase of urgent cardiac surgery patients because of cold weather or hospitals providing more accurate and timely wait time information to represent their performance for patients) and generate the corresponding results and findings by Decision Scenario Analysis Output and Decision Prediction Output. In such simulations, interesting complex emergent behavior (e.g., patient reneging patterns represented by the number of patients who left the nearest hospitals or left before being transferred by their GPs) of the cardiac surgery system is captured. Similarly, the effectiveness of adaptive resource allocation methods or strategies is evaluated by autonomous behavior-based simulations and reported by Decision Evaluation Output. By utilizing or extending the functions of 2D or 3D geographical information systems, such as Google Earth, the iHDS system in the second case employs Simulation Visualization Output to visualize the dynamics of patient arrivals and healthcare performance such as throughput, wait times and queue length, and spatial-temporal service utilization patterns, as well as the emergent behavior of the complex healthcare system for all of the above-mentioned simulations.

8.6 Remarks on the Industrial Applications of the iHDS System

Our iHDS system relates to the architecture of systems in either stand-alone, distributed, collaborative, or pervasive settings; key components of the systems and their underlying processes and couplings; the computational techniques built into the methods; input data sources integrated into and output results produced and distributed by the systems; and the modules for carrying out the corresponding user interaction, data access and collection, data integration and processing, data-driven inferences and simulation, intelligent computations, decision analytics, and support for generating solutions to various healthcare analytics and decision-making problems. The running of the iHDS system was illustrated by two working cases. One case showed how the iHDS system generated adaptive solutions for OR time block allocation. The generated output can readily be used to help ORs maintain a stable performance in the face of dynamically-changing and non-deterministic patient arrivals (e.g., due to geodemographic, environmental, climate, and socioeconomic variations). Here, the non-deterministic patients may be predicted by various statistical and mathematical techniques, although particular outcomes may not happen with complete certainty. The second case showed how the iHDS system performed decision analytics tasks and adaptive decision support in allocating regional healthcare resource, reducing healthcare performance disparities, and optimizing resource utilization.

The iHDS system may be implemented using general-purpose or specialized computing platforms, computing devices, computer processors, or electronic circuitries including, but not limited to, digital signal processors (DSP), application specific integrated circuits (ASIC), field programmable gate arrays (FPGA), and other relevant programmable logic devices configured or programmed according to the teachings of the present disclosure. Specialists can develop computer instructions or software code running on general-purpose or specialized computing platforms, computing devices, computer processors, or programmable logic devices based on the guidelines presented in this book. When implemented, the different functions of the iHDS system may be performed in a different order or concurrently with each other, if desired. Furthermore, one or more of the above-described functions may be optional or may be combined.

References

1. World Health Organization. Strengthening health systems to improve health outcomes: WHO's framework for action. 2007. http://www.who.int/healthsystems/strategy/everybodys_business.pdf. Last accessed on April 11, 2019.
2. O. Gallay. *Agent-Based Routing in Queueing Systems: Self-Organization in Production and Service Networks: From Stylized Models to Applications.* LAP Lambert Academic Publishing, 2010.
3. L.V. Bertalanffy. *General System Theory: Foundations, Development, Applications, 1st ed.* George Braziller, New York, 1969.
4. D. Katz and R.L. Kahn. *The Social Psychology of Organizations.* Wiley, 1978.
5. T.G. Cumming and C.G. Worley. *Organization Development and Change, 9th ed.* Cengage Learning, OH, USA, 2008.
6. Department of Health and Human Services Data Council, Centers for Disease Control and Prevention, National Center for Health Statistics, National Committee on Vital and Health Statistics. Shaping a health statistics vision for the 21st century. 2002. https://www.ncvhs.hhs.gov/wp-content/uploads/2014/05/21st-final-report.pdf. Last accessed on April 11, 2019.
7. L.R. Hearld, J.A. Alexander, I. Fraser, and H.J. Jiang. How do hospital organizational structure and processes affect quality of care? A critical review of research methods. *Medical Care Research and Review*, 65(3):259–299, 2008.
8. E. Warren. Final intervention report: An evidence-based approach to improving orthopedic flow and wait times. *Ottawa: Canadian Health Services Research Foundation (CHSRF)*, 2012.
9. Office of the Auditor General of Ontario. 2009 annual report: 4.09 hospitals–management and use of surgical facilities. 2009. http://www.auditor.on.ca/en/content/annualreports/arreports/en09/409en09.pdf. Last accessed on April 11, 2019.
10. Cardiac Care Network of Ontario. Access to urgent PCI for ST segment elevation myocardial infarction: Final report and recommendations. 2004. http://www.ccn.on.ca/ccn_public/UploadFiles/files/Access-To-Urgent-PCI-Final_20040705.pdf. Last accessed on August 15, 2017.
11. S.F. Lakha, B. Yegneswaran, J.C. Furlan, V. Legnini, K. Nicholson, and A. Mailis-Gagnon. Referring patients with chronic noncancer pain to pain clinics. *Canadian Family Physician*, 57(3):e106–e111, 2011.
12. D.A. Alther, T.A. Stukel, and A. Newman. The relationship between physician supply, cardiovascular health service use and cardiac disease burden in Ontario: Supply-need mismatch. *The Canadian Journal of Cardiology*, 24(3):187–193, 2008.

© Springer Nature Switzerland AG 2019
L. Tao, J. Liu, *Healthcare Service Management*, Health Information Science,
https://doi.org/10.1007/978-3-030-15385-4

13. A.J. Bagnall, S.G. Goodman, K.A. Fox, R.T. Yan, J.M. Gore, A.N. Cheema, T. Huynh, D. Chauret, D.H. Fitchett, A. Langer, and A.T. Yan. Influence of age on use of cardiac catheterization and associated outcomes in patients with non-ST-elevation acute coronary syndromes. *The American Journal of Cardiology*, 103(11):1530–1536, 2009.

14. P. Smith, J. Frank, and C. Mustard. Trends in educational inequalities in smoking and physical activity in Canada: 1974-2005. *Journal of Epidemiology and Community Health*, 63:317–323, 2009.

15. A. Tramarin, S. Campostrini, K. Tolley, and F.D. Lalla. The influence of socioeconomic status on health service utilisation by patients with AIDS in North Italy. *British Journal of Clinical Pharmacology*, 45(6):859–866, 1997.

16. N.A. Christakis and J.H. Fowler. The spread of obesity in a large social network over 32 years. *The New England Journal of Medicine*, 257:370–379, 2007.

17. R. Chunara, L. Bouton, J.W. Ayers, and J.S. Brownstein. Assessing the online social environment for surveillance of obesity prevalence. *PLoS ONE*, 8(4), 2013.

18. Ontario Ministry of Finance. Long-term sustainability of Ontario public services. In *Ontario's Long-Term Report on the Economy*, pages 43–54, 2010. http://www.fin.gov.on.ca/en/economy/ltr/2010/. Last accessed on April 11, 2019.

19. J. Mackay and G. Mensah. *The Atlas of Heart Disease and Strokes*. World Health Organization, Geneva, 2004.

20. D.A. Alter, E.A. Cohen, W. Wang, K.W. Glasgow, P.M. Slaughter, and J.V. Tu. Cardiac procedures. In *Access to Health Services in Ontario*, 2nd., J.V. Tu, S.P. Pinfold, P. McColgan, and A. Laupacis, eds., Institute for Clinical Evaluative Sciences, Ontario, 2006. https://www.ices.on.ca/Publications/Atlases-and-Reports/2006/Access-to-health-services-2nd-ed. Last accessed on April 11, 2019.

21. J.E. Seidel, C.A. Beck, G. Pocobelli, J.B. Lemaire, J.M. Bugar, and H. Quan. Location of residence associated with the likelihood of patient visit to the preoperative assessment clinic. *BMC health services research*, 6:13, 2006.

22. S.L. Grace, A. Evindar, B.L. Abramson, and D.E. Stewart. Physician management preferences for cardiac patients: Factors affecting referral to cardiac rehabilitation. *The Canadian Journal of Cardiology*, 20(11):1101–1107, 2004.

23. Institute of Medicine. *The Future of the Public's Health in the 21st Century*. The National Academies Press, Washington, DC, 2003.

24. B. Barua and N. Esmail. Waiting your turn: Wait times for health care in Canada. 2012. https://www.fraserinstitute.org/sites/default/files/waiting-your-turn-2012-rev.pdf. Last accessed on April 11, 2019.

25. K. Resnicow and E.P. Page. Embracing chaos and complexity: A quantum change for public health. *American Journal of Public Health*, 98(8):1382–1389, 2008.

26. W.B. Rouse. Health care as a complex adaptive system: Implications for design and management. *The Bridge*, 38(1):17–25, 2008.

27. L.A. Lipsitz. Understanding health care as a complex system: The foundation for unintended consequences. *The Journal of the American Medical Association*, 308(3):243–244, 2012.

28. Cardiac Care Network of Ontario. Patient, physician and Ontario household survey reports: Executive summaries. http://www.ccn.on.ca/ccn_public/uploadfiles/files/ccn_survey_exec_sum_200508.pdf. 2005. Last accessed on August 15, 2017.

29. H.C. Wijeysundera, T.A. Stukel, A. Chong, M.K. Natarajan, and D.A. Alter. Impact of clinical urgency, physician supply and procedural capacity on regional variations in wait times for coronary angiography. *BMC Health Services Research*, 10:5, 2010.

30. H.A. Simon. Bounded rationality and organizational learning. *Organization Science*, 2(1):125–134, 1991.

31. H.R. Priesmeyer and L.F. Sharp. Phase plane analysis: Applying chaos theory in health care. *Quality Management in Health Care*, 4(1):62–70, 1995.

32. H.R. Priesmeyer, L.F. Sharp, L. Wammack, and J.D. Mabrey. Chaos theory and clinical pathways: A practical application. *Quality Management in Health Care*, 4(4):63–72, 1996.

33. M. Arndt and B. Bigelow. Commentary: The potential of chaos theory and complexity theory for health services management. *Health Care Management Review*, 25(1):35–38, 2000.
34. J.W. Begun and K.R. White. The profession of nursing as a complex adaptive system: Strategies for change. *Research in the Sociology of Health Care*, 16:189–203, 1999.
35. D.P. Smethurst and H.C. Williams. Self-regulation in hospital waiting lists. *Journal of the Royal Society of Medicine*, 95:287–289, 2002.
36. J. Liu, X. Jin, and K.C. Tsui. *Autonomy Oriented Computing: From Problem Solving to Complex Systems Modeling*. Kluwer Academic Publishers, New York, 2004.
37. Institute of Medicine (US) Committee on Health and Behavior: Research, Practice, and Policy. Individuals and families: Models and interventions. In *Health and Behavior: The Interplay of Biological, Behavioral, and Societal Influences*. Washington (DC): National Academies Press (US), 2001. http://www.ncbi.nlm.nih.gov/books/NBK43749/. Last accessed on April 11, 2019.
38. J.J. Mira, S. Lorenzo, and I. Navarro. Hospital reputation and perceptions of patient safety. *Medical Principle and Practice*, 23(1):92–94, 2014.
39. D.P. Smethurst and H.C. Williams. Are hospital waiting lists self-regulating? *Nature*, 410:652–653, 2001.
40. S.B. Buchbinder and N.H. Shanks. *Introduction to Health Care Management, Second Edition*. Jones and Bartlett Learning, MA, 2011.
41. World Health Organization. Building leadership and management capacity in health. 2007. http://www.who.int/management/FrameworkBrochure.pdf. Last accessed on April 11, 2019.
42. T. Schoenmeyr, P.F. Dunn, D. Gamarnik, R. Levi, D.L. Berger, B.J. Daily, W.C. Levine, and W.S. Sandberg. A model for understanding the impacts of demand and capacity on waiting time to enter a congested recovery room. *Anesthesiology*, 110:1293–1304, 2009.
43. P.I. Buerhaus, D.O. Staiger, and D.I. Auerbach. *The Future of the Nursing Workforce in the United States: Data, Trends, and Implications*. Jones and Bartlett Publishers, Boston, MA, 2009.
44. J. Liu, L. Tao, and B. Xiao. Discovering the impact of preceding units' characteristics on the wait time of cardiac surgery unit from statistic data. *PLoS One*, 6(7):e21959, 2011.
45. L. Tao, J. Liu, and B. Xiao. Effects of geodemographic profiles on healthcare service utilization: A case study on cardiac care in Ontario, Canada. *BMC Health Services Research*, 13:239, 2013.
46. M. Knapman and A. Bonner. Overcrowding in medium-volume emergency departments: Effects of aged patients in emergency departments on wait times for non-emergent triage-level patients. *International Journal of Nursing Practice*, 16:310–317, 2010.
47. C. Sanmartin, J.M. Merthelot, and C.N. Mcintosh. Determinants of unacceptable waiting times for specialized services in Canada. *Healthcare Policy*, 2(3):e140–e154, 2007.
48. J.F. Hair, R.E. Anderson, R.L. Tatham, and W.C. Black. *Multivariate Data Analysis: With Readings, 5th ed.* Pearson Prentice Hall, Englewood Cliffs, NJ, 1998.
49. R. Liu, L. So, S. Mohan, N. Khan, K. King, and H. Quan. Cardiovascular risk factors in ethnic populations within Canada: Results from national cross-sectional surveys. *Open Medicine*, 4(3):E143, 2010.
50. J. Li, L. Guo, and N. Handly. Hospital admission prediction using pre-hospital variables. In *Proceedings of the 2009 IEEE International Conference on Bioinformatics and Biomedicine, Washington D.C., USA*, pages 283–286, 2009.
51. M.L. McCarthy, S.L. Zeger, R. Ding, D. Aronsky, N.R. Hoot, and G.D. Kelen. The challenge of predicting demand for emergency department services. *Academic Emergency Medicine*, 15:337–346, 2008.
52. P. Yi, S.K. George, J.A. Paul, and L. Lin. Hospital capacity planning for disaster emergency management. *Socio-Economic Planning Sciences*, 44:151–160, 2010.
53. A. Ercole, D.K. Menon, and D.R. O'Donnell. Modelling the impact of pandemic influenza A(H1N1) on UK paediatric intensive care demand. *Archives of Disease in Childhood*, 94:962–964, 2009.

54. S. Fomundam and J. Herrmann. A survey of queuing theory applications in healthcare. Technical report, The Institute for Systems Research, University of Maryland, 2007.

55. S.H. Jacobson, S.N. Hall, and J.R. Swisher. Application of discrete-event simulation in health care clinics: A survey. In *Patient Flow: Reducing Delay in Healthcare Delivery*, pages 211–252. Springer, R.W. Hall, eds., Springer, New York, 2006.

56. I. Ozkarahan. Allocation of surgical procedures to operating rooms. *Journal of Medical Systems*, 19(4):333–352, 1995.

57. P.E. Plsek and T. Greenhalgh. The challenge of complexity in health care. *BMJ*, 323:625–628, 2001.

58. The Complex Systems Modeling Group (CSMG). *Modeling in Healthcare*. American Mathematical Society, 2010.

59. K.E. Maani and R.Y. Cavana. *Systems Thinking, System Dynamics: Managing Change and Complexity*. Prentice Hall, Auckland, NZ, 2000.

60. Paranjape, R. and Sadanand, A. *Multi-Agent Systems for Healthcare Simulation and Modeling: Applications for System Improvement*. IGI Global, 2009.

61. D. Gefen, D.W. Straub, and M.C. Boudreau. Structural equation modeling and regression: Guidelines for research practice. *Communications of the Association for Information Systems*, 4:7, 2000.

62. D.W. Gerbing and J.C. Anderson. An updated paradigm for scale development incorporating unidimensionality and its assessment. *Journal of Marketing Research*, 25:186–192, 1988.

63. L. Liu. Autonomy-Oriented Computing: The nature and implications of a paradigm for self-organized computing. In *Proceedings of the Fourth International Conference on Natural Computation, and the Fifth International Conference on Fuzzy Systems and Knowledge Discovery*, pages 3–11, 2008.

64. J. Liu. *Autonomous Agents and Multi-Agent Systems: Explorations in Learning, Self-Organization and Adaptive Computation*. World Scientific Publishing, Singapore, 2001.

65. Cardiac Care Network of Ontario. Cardiac surgery in Ontario: Ensuring continued excellence and leadership in patient care. 2006. http://www.ccn.on.ca/ccn_public/uploadfiles/files/Surgical_Report_October31_2006_BOARD.pdf. Last accessed on August 15, 2016.

66. K.A. Wager, F.W. Lee, and J.P. Glaser. *Health Care Information Systems: A Practical Approach for Health Care Management, 2nd ed.* Jossey-Bass, San Francisco, CA, 2009.

67. Institute of Medicine. *Clinical Data as the Basic Staple of Health Learning: Creating and Protecting a Public Good: Workshop Summary*. The National Academies Press, Washington, DC, 2010.

68. Ontario Ministry of Finance. 2006 census highlights. http://www.fin.gov.on.ca/en/economy/demographics/census/cenhi06-1.html. Last accessed on April 11, 2019.

69. Cardiac Care Network of Ontario. Cardiac care network: Annual report 11-12. 2012. http://www.ccn.on.ca/ccn_public/uploadfiles/files/CCN_Annual_Report_2012.pdf. Last accessed on August 15, 2017.

70. L. Bertalanffy. *General System Theory: Foundations, Development, Applications*. George Braziller, New York, 1969.

71. P.V. Asaro, L.M. Lewis, and S.B. Boxerman. The impact of input and output factors on emergency department throughput. *Academic Emergency Medicine*, 14:235–242, 2007.

72. G.C. Harewood, H. Ryan, F. Murray, and S. Patchett. Potential impact of enhanced practice efficiency on endoscopy waiting times. *IRISH Journal of Medical Science*, 178(2):187–192, 2009.

73. C.E. Kim, J.-S. Shin, J. Lee, Y.J. Lee, M. Kim, A. Choi, K.B. Park, H.-J. Lee, and I.-H. Ha. Quality of medical service, patient satisfaction and loyalty with a focus on interpersonal-based medical service encounters and treatment effectiveness: a cross-sectional multicenter study of complementary and alternative medicine (cam) hospitals. *BMC Complementary and Alternative Medicine*, 17(1):174, 2017.

74. I.T. Jolliffe. *Principal Component Analysis, 2nd ed.* Springer, New York, 2002.

75. N. Saint-Jacques, T. Younis, R. Dewar, and D. Rayson. Wait times for breast cancer care. *British Journal of Cancer*, 96(1):162–168, 2007.

76. D.I.M.S. Pillay, R.J.D.M Ghazali, N.H.A. Manaf, A.H.A. Abdullah, A.A. Bakar, F. Salikin, M. Umapathy, R. Ali, N. Bidin, and W.I.W. Ismail. Hospital waiting time: The forgotten premise of healthcare service delivery? *International Journal of Health Care Quality Assurance*, 24(7):506–522, 2011.

77. M.S. Westaway, P. Rheeder, D.G.V. Zyl, and J.R. Seager. Interpersonal and organizational dimensions of patient satisfaction: The moderating effects of health status. *International Journal for Quality in Health Care*, 15(4):337–344, 2003.

78. S. Löfendahl, I. Eckerlund, H. Hansagi, B. Malmqvist, S. Resch, and M. Hanning. Waiting for orthopedic surgery: Factors associated with waiting times and patients' opinion. *International Journal for Quality in Health Care*, 17(2):133–140, 2005.

79. S.W. Menard. *Logistic Regression Analysis: From Introductory to Advanced Concepts and Applications*. SAGE Publications, Thousand Oaks, CA, 2009.

80. J.E. Klein-Geltink, L.M. Pogany, R.D. Barr, M.L. Greenberg, and L.S. Mery. Waiting times for cancer care in Canadian children: Impact of distance, clinical, and demographic factors. *Pediatric Blood and Cancer*, 44(4):318–327, 2005.

81. S.J. Aragon and S.B. Gesell. A patient satisfaction theory and its robustness across gender in emergency departments: A multigroup structural equation modeling investigation. *American Journal of Medical Quality*, 18(6):229–241, 2003.

82. C.J. Chiu, L.A. Wray, E.A. Beverly, and O.G. Dominic. The role of health behaviors in mediating the relationship between depressive symptoms and glycemic control in type 2 diabetes: A structural equation modeling approach. *Social Psychiatry and Psychiatric Epidemiology*, 45(1):67–76, 2010.

83. P.A. Heidenreich, J.G. Trogdon, O.A. Khavjou, J. Butler, K. Dracup, and et al. Forecasting the future of cardiovascular disease in the United States. *Circulation*, 123:933–944, 2011.

84. G. Dunn, M. Mirandola, F. Amaddeo, and M. Tansella. Describing, explaining or predicting mental health care costs: A guide to regression models: Methodological review. *The Bristish Journal of Psychiatry: The Journal of Mental Science*, 183:398–404, 2003.

85. C.A. Hubera, S. Schneeweissb, A. Signorella, and O. Reicha. Improved prediction of medical expenditures and health care utilization using an updated chronic disease score and claims data. *Journal of Clinical Epidemiology*, 66(10):1118–1127, 2013.

86. P.F. Dunn. *Measurement and Data Analysis for Engineering and Science*. McGraw-Hill, New York, 2005.

87. M.C. Spaeder and J.C. Fackler. Time series model to predict burden of viral respiratory illness on a pediatric intensive care unit. *Medical Decision Making*, 31(3):494–499, 2011.

88. M.H. Hassan, A.A. Zaghloul, and S.A. Mokhtar. The probability distribution of attendance to hospital emergency units for school students in Alexandria. *The Journal of the Egyptian Public Health Association*, 80(1-2):127–151, 2005.

89. Y.A. Ozcan. *Quantitative Methods in Health Care Management: Techniques and Applications, 2nd ed.* Jossey-Bass, San Francisco, 2009.

90. D. Gross, J.F. Shortle, J.M. Thompson, and C.M. Harris. *Fundamentals of Queueing Theory*. Wiley, Hoboken, NJ, 2009.

91. D.W. Strooc. *An Introduction to Markov Processes*. Springer, New York, 2005.

92. S. Palaniammal. *Probability and Queueing Theory*. PHI Learning Private Limited, New Delhi, 2012.

93. W. England and S. Roberts. Applications of computer simulation in health care. In *Proceedings of the 1978 Winter Simulation Conference, Institute of Electrical and Electronics Engineers, Florida, USA*, pages 665–676, 1978.

94. G.S. Fishman. *Discrete-Event Simulation: Modeling, Programming, and Analysis*. Springer, New York, 2001.

95. L.M. Leemis and S.K. Park. *Discrete-Event Simulation: A First Course*. Pearson Prentice Hall, Upper Saddle River, NJ, 2006.

96. S. Creemers and M. Lambrecht. Healthcare queueing models. Technical report, Katholieke Universiteit Leuven, 2008. http://www.stefancreemers.be/PDF/KBI_0804.pdf. Last accessed on April 11, 2019.

97. J. Jun, S.H. Jacobson, and J.R. Swisher. Application of discrete-event simulation in health care clinics: A survey. *Journal of the Operational Research Society*, 50(2):109–123, 1999.

98. D. Fone, Temple M. Hollinghurst, S., A. Round, N. Lester, A. Weightman, K. Roberts, E. Coyle, G. Bevan, and S. Palmer. Systematic review of the use and value of computer simulation modelling in population health and health care delivery. *Journal of Public Health Medicine*, 25(4):325–335, 2003.

99. M.M. Günal and M. Pidd. Discrete event simulation for performance modelling in health care: A review of the literature. *European Journal of Operational Research*, 4:42–51, 2010.

100. B. Cardoen, E. Demeulemeester, and J. Belien. Operating room planning and scheduling: A literature review. *European Journal of Operational Research*, 201(3):921–932, 2010.

101. J.W. Forrester. *Urban Dynamics*. MIT Press, Cambridge, Mass, 1969.

102. J.B. Homer and G.B. Hirsch. System dynamics modeling for public health: Background and opportunities. *American Journal of Public Health*, 92:452–458, 2006.

103. S.C. Brailsford, V.A. Lattimer, P. Tarnaras, and J.C. Turnbull. Emergency and on-demand health care: Modelling a large complex system. *Journal of the Operational Research Society*, 55:34–42, 2004.

104. R. Diaz, J.G. Behr, and M. Tulpule. A system dynamics model for simulating ambulatory health care demands. *Simulation in Healthcare: Journal of the Society for Simulation in Healthcare*, 7(4):243–250, 2012.

105. V. Grimm and S.F. Railsback. *Individual-Based Modeling and Ecology*. Princeton University Press, New Jersey, 2005.

106. J. Neumann. *Theory of Self-Reproducing Automata*. University of Illinois Press, Urbana and London, 1966.

107. M. Gardner. Mathematical games: The fantastic combinations of John Conway's new solitaire game "life". *Scientific American*, 223:120–123, 1970.

108. M. Wooldridge. *An Introduction to Multi-Agent Systems*. John Wiley & Sons, New York, 2009.

109. E. Bonabeau. Agent-based modeling: Methods and techniques for simulating human systems. *Proceedings of the National Academy of Sciences of the United States of American*, 99(Suppl. 3):7280–7287, 2002.

110. J.M. Epstein. *Generative Social Science: Studies in Agent-Based Computational Modeling*. Princeton University Press, Princeton, NJ, 2006.

111. A. Ghorbani, P. Bots, V. Dianum, and G. Dijkema. Maia: A framework for developing agent-based social simulations. *Journal of Artificial Societies and Social Simulation*, 16(2):9, 2013.

112. S.C. Bankes. Agent-based modeling: A revolution? *Proceedings of the National Academy of Sciences of the United States of America*, 99:7199, 2002.

113. C.M. Macal and M.J. North. Tutorial on agent-based modelling and simulation. *Journal of Simulation*, 4:151–162, 2010.

114. V. Grimm, U. Berger, F. Bastiansen, S. Eliassen, V. Ginot, J. Giske, and etc. A standard protocol for describing individual-based and agent-based models. *Ecological Modeling*, 198:115–126, 2006.

115. V. Grimm and S.F. Railsback. Pattern-oriented modeling: A 'multi-scope' for predictive systems ecology. *Philosophical Transactions of The Royal Society B*, 367(1586):298–310, 2012.

116. P.S. Andrews, F.A.C. Polack, A.T. Sampson, S. Stepney, and J. Timmis. The CoSMoS process, version 0.1: A process for the modelling and simulation of complex systems. Technical report, Department of Computer Science, University of York, 2010.

117. V. Grimm, E. Revilla, U. Berger, F. Jeltsch, W.M. Mooij, S.F. Railsback, H.H. Thulke, J. Weiner, T. Wiegand, and D.L. DeAngelis. Pattern-oriented modeling of agent-based complex systems: Lessons from ecology. *Science*, 310:987–991, 2005.

118. S.F. Railsback and M.D. Johnson. Pattern-oriented modeling of bird foraging and pest control in coffee farms. *Ecological Modelling*, 222:3305–3319, 2011.

119. L. Leykum, P. Kumar, M. Parchman, R.R. McDaniel, H. Lanham, and M. Agar. Use of an agent-based model to understand clinical systems. *Journal of Artificial Societies and Social Simulation*, 15(3):2, 2012.

120. S. Eubank, H. Guclu, V.S.A. Kumar, M.V. Marathe, A. Srinivasan, Z. Toroczkai, and N. Wang. Modelling disease outbreaks in realistic urban social networks. *Nature*, 429:180–184, 2004.

121. B. Ajelli, M. Goncalves, D. Balcan, V. Colizza, H. Hu, J.J. Ramasco, S. Merler, and A. Vespignani. Comparing large-scale computational approaches to epidemic modeling: Agent-based versus structured metapopulation models. *BMC Infectious Diseases*, 10:190, 2010.

122. S. Barnes, B. Golden, and S. Price. Applications of agent-based modeling and simulation to healthcare operations management. *Handbook of Healthcare Operations Management: Methods and Applications*, 184:45–74, 2013.

123. A.K. Hutzschenreuter, P.A.N. Bosman, I. Blonk-Altena, J. Aarle, and Poutré. Agent-based patient admission scheduling in hospitals. In *Proceedings of the Twelfth International Conference on Autonomous Agents and Multiagent Systems*, 2008.

124. S. Zhang and J. Liu. A massively multi-agent system for discovering HIV-immune interaction dynamics. *Lecture Notes in Computer Science*, 3446:161–173, 2005.

125. F.A. Spencer, R.J. Goldberg, P.D. Frederick, J. Malmgren, R.C. Becker, and J.M. Gore. Age and the utilization of cardiac catheterization following uncomplicated first acute myocardial infarction treated with thrombolytic therapy (The Second National Registry of Myocardial Infarction [NRMI-2]). *The American Journal of Cardiology*, 88(2):107–111, 2001.

126. M.A. Winkleby, D.E. Jatulis, E. Frank, and S.P. Fortmann. Socioeconomic status and health: How education, income, and occupation contribute to risk factors for cardiovascular disease. *American Journal of Public Health*, 82:816–820, 1992.

127. M.A. Winkleby, H.C. Kraemer, D.K. Ahn, and A.N. Varady. Ethnic and socioeconomic differences in cardiovascular disease risk factors: Findings for women from the third national health and nutrition examination survey, 1988-1994. *Journal of the American Medical Association*, 280(4):356–362, 1998.

128. Ontario Ministry of Finance. *Ontario Population Projections Update, 2010-2036*. Queen's Printer for Ontario, 2011.

129. S.E. Bronskill, M.W. Carter, A.P. Costa, A.V. Esensoy, S.S. Gill, A. Gruneir, D.A. Henry, J.P. Hirdes, R.L. Jaakkimainen, J.W. Poss, and W.P. Wodchis. Aging in Ontario: An ICES Chartbook of Health Service Use by Older Adults. 2010. https://www.ices.on.ca/Publications/ Atlases-and-Reports/2010/Aging-in-Ontario. Last accessed on April 11, 2019.

130. T. McIntosh, M. Ducie, M.B. Charles, J. Church, J. Lavis, M.P. Pomey, N. Smith, and S. Tomblin. Population health and health system reform: Needs-based funding for health services in five provinces. *Canadian Political Science Review*, 4(1):42–61, 2010.

131. A. Alguwaihes and B.R. Shah. Educational attainment is associated with health care utilization and self-care behavior by individuals with diabetes. *The Open Diabetes Journal*, 2:24–28, 2009.

132. J.B. Strom and P. Libby. Atherosclerosis. In *Pathophysiology of Heart Disease: A Collaborative Project of Medical Students and Faculty, 5th ed.*, pages 113–134, L.S. Lilly, eds., Lippincott Williams and Wilkins, New York, 2010.

133. E.G. Lakatta. Age-associated cardiovascular changes in health: Impact on cardiovascular disease in older persons. *Heart Failure Reviews*, 7(1):29–49, 2002.

134. C.M. Chow, L. Donovan, D. Manuel, H. Johansen, and J.V. Tu. Regional variation in self-reported heart disease prevalence in Canada. *The Canadian Journal of Cardiology*, 21(14):1265–1271, 2005.

135. A. Grover, K. Gorman, T.M. Dall, R. Jonas, B. Lytle, R. Shemin, D. Wood, and I. Kron. Shortage of cardiothoracic surgeons is likely by 2020. *Circulation*, 120(6):488–494, 2009.

136. Cardiac Care Network of Ontario. Cardiac care network moving forward: Annual report 07-08. 2008. http://www.ccn.on.ca/ccn_public/UploadFiles/files/CCN%202007-2008 %20Annual%20Report.pdf. Last accessed on August 15, 2017.

137. P. Apparicio, M. Abdelmajid, M. Riva, and R. Shearmur. Comparing alternative approaches to measuring the geographical accessibility of urban health services: Distance types and aggregation-error issues. *International Journal of Health Geographics*, 7:7, 2008.

138. E.M. Bosanac, R.C. Parkinson, and D.S. Hall. Geographic access to hospital care: A 30-minute travel time standard. *Medical Care*, 14(7):616–624, 1976.
139. L. Chan, L.G. Hart, and D.C. Goodman. Geographic access to health care for rural medicare beneficiaries. *The Journal of Rural Health*, 22:140–146, 2006.
140. N. Suskin, S. MacDonald, T. Swabey, H. Arthur, M.A. Vimr, and R. Tihaliani. Cardiac rehabilitation and secondary prevention services in Ontario: Recommendations from a consensus panel. *The Canadian Journal of Cardiology*, 19:833–838, 2003.
141. L. Wang. Analysing spatial accessibility to health care: A case study of access by different immigrant groups to primary care physicians in Toronto. *Annals of GIS*, 17(4):237–251, 2011.
142. N. Schuurman, N.J. Bell, R. L'Heureux, and S.M. Hameed. Modeling optimal location for pre-hospital helicopter emergency medical services. *BMC Emergency Medicine*, 9:6, 2009.
143. T. Coltman, T.M. Devinney, D.F. Midgley, and S. Venaik. Formative versus reflective measurement models: Two applications of formative measurement. *Journal of Business Research*, 61:1250–1262, 2008.
144. C. Fornell. A second generation of multivariate analysis: Classification of methods and implications for marketing research. In *Review of Marketing*, pages 407–450, M.J. Houston, eds., American Marketing Association, 1987.
145. S. Petrou and J. Wolstenholme. A review of alternative approaches to healthcare resource allocation. *Pharmacoeconomics*, 18:33–43, 2000.
146. G. Kephart and Y. Asada. Need-based resource allocation: Different need indicator, different result? *BMC Health Service Research*, 9:122, 2009.
147. J. Blanden and P. Gregg. Family income and educational attainment: A review of approaches and evidence for britain. *Oxford Review of Economic Policy*, 20(2):245–263, 2004.
148. D. Fusco, C. Saitto, M. Arcà, and C.A. Perucci. Cyclic fluctuations in hospital bed occupancy in Roma (Italy): Supply or demand driven? *Health Service Management Research*, 16(4):268–275, 2003.
149. E.P. Jack and T.L. Powers. A review and synthesis of demand management, capacity management and performance in health-care services. *International Journal of Management Reviews*, 11(2):149–174, 2009.
150. P. Deb and P.K. Trivedi. Demand for medical care by the elderly in the United States: A finite mixture approach. *Journal of Applied Econometrics*, 12:313–336, 1997.
151. W. Pohlmeier and V. Ulrich. An econometric model of the two-part decisionmaking process in the demand for health care. *The Journal of Human Resources*, 30:339–361, 1995.
152. N. Duan, W.G. Manning, C.N. Morris, and J.P. Newhouse. A comparison of alternative models for the demand for medical care. *Journal of Business and Economic Statistics*, 1:115–126, 1983.
153. W.G. Manning, J.P. Newhouse, N. Duan, E.B. Keeler, A. Leibowitz, and M.S. Marquis. Health insurance and the demand for medical care: Evidence from a randomized experiment. *American Economic Review*, 77:251–277, 1987.
154. P. Hossain, B. Kawar, and M.E. Nahas. Obesity and diabetes in the developing world – A growing challenge. *The New England Journal of Medicine*, 356:213–215, 2007.
155. D.J. Heaney, J.G. Howie, and A.M. Porter. Factors influencing waiting times and consultation times in general practice. *The British Journal of General Practice*, 41(349):315–319, 1991.
156. C.M. Blanchard, R.D. Reid, L. Morrin, L. McDonnell, K. McGannon, R. Rhodes, J. Spence, and N. Edwards. Demographic and clinical determinants of moderate to vigorous physical activity during home-based cardiac rehabilitation: The home-based determinants of exercise (HOME) study. *Journal of Cardiopulmonary Rehabilitation & Prevention*, 30(4):240–245, 2010.
157. E. Odubanjo, K. Bennett, and J. Feely. Influence of socioeconomic status on the quality of prescribing in the elderly – A population based study. *British Journal of Clinical Pharmacology*, 58(5):496–502, 2004.
158. A. Marshall, C. Vasilakis, and E. El-Darzi. Length of stay-based patient flow models: Recent developments and future directions. *Health Care Management Science*, 8(3):213–220, 2005.

159. D. Bamford and E. Chatziaslan. Healthcare capacity measurement. *International Journal of Productivity and Performance Management*, 58(8):748–766, 2010.

160. J.J. Pandit, M. Pandit, and J.M. Reynard. Understanding waiting lists as the matching of surgical capacity to demand: Are we wasting enough surgical time? *Anaesthesia*, 65(6):625–640, 2010.

161. *The Reform of Health Care Systems: A Review of Seventeen OECD Countries*. Organisation for Economic Co-operation and Development, Paris, 1994.

162. R.M. Rosser. A health index and output measure. In *Quality of Life Assessment: Key Issues in the 1990s*, pages 151–178, S.R. Walker and R.M. Rosser, eds., Kluwer Academic Publishers, 1993.

163. D.A. Alter, E.A. Cohen, G. Cernat, K.W. Glasgow, P.M. Slaughter, and J.V. Tu. Cardiac procedures. In *Access to Health Services in Ontario*, 1st ed., J.V. Tu, S.P. Pinfold, P. McColgan, and A. Laupacis, eds., Institute for Clinical Evaluative Sciences, 2005. https://www.ices.on.ca/Publications/Atlases-and-Reports/2005/Access-to-health-services. Last accessed on April 11, 2019.

164. A.V. Ackere and P.C. Smith. Towards a macro model of national health service waiting lists. *System Dynamics Review*, 15(3):225–252, 1999.

165. R.F. Davies. Waiting lists for health care: A necessary evil. *Canadian Medical Association*, 160(10):1469–1470, 1999.

166. A. Basinski, D. Almond, R.G.G. James, and C.D. Naylor. Rating the urgency of coronary angiography: Results of an expert panel process. *The Canadian Journal of Cardiology*, 9(4):313–321, 1993.

167. C.D. Naylor, R.S. Baigrie, B.S. Goldman, J.A. Cairns, D.S. Beanlands, and N. Berman. Assigning priority to patients requiring coronary revascularization: Consensus principles from a panel of cardiologists and cardiac surgeons. *The Canadian Journal of Cardiology*, 7(5):207–213, 1991.

168. L.C. Baker. The challenges of health system capacity growth. Technical report, The National Institute for Health Care Management Research and Educational Foundation, 2008. http://www.nihcm.org/pdf/CapacityBrief-FINAL.pdf. Last accessed on April 11, 2019.

169. S. Trzeciak and E.P. Rivers. Emergency department overcrowding in the United States: An emerging threat to patient safety and public health. *American Journal of Medical Quality*, 20:402–405, 2003.

170. A. Brenner, Z. Zeng, Y. Liu, J. Wang, J. Li, and P.K. Howard. Modeling and analysis of the emergency department at University of Kentucky Chandler Hospital using simulations. *Journal of Emergency Nursing*, 36:303–310, 2010.

171. L. Kosnik. Breakthrough demand-capacity management strategies to improve hospital flow, safety, and satisfaction. In *Patient Flow: Reducing Delay in Healthcare Delivery*, pages 101–122, R.W. Hall, eds., Springer, 2006.

172. Canadian Institute for Health Information. Waiting for health care in Canada: What we know and what we don't know. 2006. https://secure.cihi.ca/estore/productSeries.htm?pc=PCC311. Last accessed on April 11, 2019.

173. E.A. Antman, D.T. Anbe, P.W. Armstrong, E.R. Bates, L.A. Green, M. Hand, J.S. Hochman, and H.M. Krumholz. ACC/AHA guidelines for the management of patients with ST-Elevation myocardial infarction-executive summary. *Circulation*, 110:588–636, 2004.

174. D.A. Alter, P. Austin, and J.V. Tu. Use of coronary angiography, angioplasty and bypass surgery after acute myocardial infarction in Ontario. In *Cardiovascular Health and Services in Ontario: An ICES Atlas*, pages 141–164, D. Naylor and P. Slaughter, eds., ICES Atlas, 1999. https://www.ices.on.ca/Publications/Atlases-and-Reports/1999/Cardiovascular-health-and-services. Last accessed on April 11, 2019.

175. F.L. Lucas, A.E. Siewers, D.J. Malenka, and D.E. Wennberg. The diagnostic-therapeutic cascade revisited: Coronary angiography, CABG and PCI in the modern era. *Circulation*, 118(25):2797–2802, 2008.

176. D. Verrilli and H.G. Welch. The impact of diagnostic testing in therapeutic interventions. *The Journal of the American Medical Association*, 275:1189–1191, 1996.

177. D.E. Wennberg, J.D.J. Dickens, L. Biener, F.J. Fowler, D.N. Soule, and R.B. Keller. Do physicians do what they say? The inclination to test and its association with coronary angiography rates. *Journal of General Internal Medicine*, 12:172–176, 1997.

178. Institute for Clinical Evaluative Sciences. Report on coronary artery bypass surgery in Ontario, fiscal years 2005/06 and 2006/07. 2008. https://www.ices.on.ca/Publications/Atlases-and-Reports/2008/Report-on-coronary-artery-bypass-surgery. Last accessed on April 11, 2019.

179. R. Hughes and D. Lee. Using data describing physician inpatient practice patterns: Issues and opportunities. *Health Care Management Review*, 16(1):33–40, 1991.

180. P.I. Buerhaus. Current and future state of the US nursing workforce. *The Journal of the American Medical Association*, 300(20):2422–2424, 2008.

181. J.E. Justman, S. Koblavi-Deme, A. Tanuri, A. Goldberg, L.F. Gonzalez, and C.R. Gwynn. HIV scale-up and global health systems. *Journal of Acquired Immune Deficiency Syndromes*, 52:s30–s33, 2009.

182. R.P. Freckleton and W.J. Sutherland. Do power laws imply self-regulation? *Nature*, 413:382, 2001.

183. A.K. Mukherjee. A simulation model for management of operations in the pharmacy of a hospital. *Simulation*, 56(2):91–103, 1991.

184. J. Patrick, M. Puterman, and M. Queyranne. Dynamic multi-priority patient scheduling for a diagnostic resource. *Operations Research*, 56(5):1507–1525, 2008.

185. P. Santibáñez, V.S. Chow, J. French, M.L. Puterman, and S. Tyldesley. Reducing patient wait times and improving resource utilization at British Columbia cancer agency's ambulatory care unit through simulation. *Health Care Management Science*, 12(4):392–407, 2009.

186. S. Willcox, M. Seddon, S. Dunn, R.T. Edwards, J. Pearse, and J.V. Tu. Measuring and reducing waiting times: A cross-national comparison of strategies. *Health Affairs*, 26(4):1078–1087, 2007.

187. C. Fornell and F. Bookstein. Two structural equation models: LISREL and PLS applied to consumer exit-voice theory. *Journal of Marketing Research*, 19:440–452, 1982.

188. S.M. Friedman, L. Schofield, and S. Tirkos. Do as I say, not as I do: A survey of public impressions of queue-jumping and preferential access. *European Journal of Emergency Medicine*, 14:260–264, 2007.

189. K.P. Unnikrishnan, D. Patnaik, and T.J. Iwashyna. Discovering specific cascades in critical care transfer networks. In *Proceedings of the First ACM International Health Informatics Symposium, Arlington, Virginia, USA*, pages 541–544, 2010.

190. J.H. Heijmans, J.G. Maessen, and P.M.H.J. Poekaerts. Risk stratification for adverse outcome in cardiac surgery. *European Journal of Anaesthesiology*, 20:515–527, 2003.

191. F. Immer, J. Habicht, K. Nessensohn, F. Bernet, P. Stulz, M. Kaufmann, and K. Skarvan. Prospective evaluation of 3 risk stratification scores in cardiac surgery. *Thoracic and Cardiovascular Surgery*, 48:134–139, 2000.

192. L. Ridderstolpe, H. Gill, M. Borga, H. Rutberg, and H. Ahlfeldt. Canonical correlation analysis of risk factors and clinical outcomes in cardiac surgery. *Journal of Medical Systems*, 29(4):357–377, 2005.

193. S. Burke. Missing values, outliers, robust statistics & non-parametric methods. *LCGC Europe Online Supplement*, 59:19–24, 2001.

194. G.E.A.P.A. Batista and M.C. Monard. An analysis of four missing data treatment methods for supervised learning. *Applied Artificial Intelligence: An International Journal*, 17(5 & 6):519–533, 2003.

195. A.A. Ray, K.J. Buth, J.A. Sullivan, D.E. Johnstone, and G.M. Hirsch. Waiting for cardiac surgery: Results of a risk-stratified queuing process. *Circulation*, 104:I92–I98, 2001.

196. C.D. Naylor, K. Sykora, S.B. Jaglal, S. Jefferson, and the Steering Committee of the Adult Cardiac Care Network of Ontario. Waiting for coronary artery bypass surgery: Population-based study of 8517 consecutive patients in Ontario, Canada. *Lancet*, 346:1605–1609, 1995.

197. C.D. Naylor, C.D. Morgan, C.M. Levinton, S. Wheeler, L. Hunter, K. Klymciw, R.S. Baigrie, and B.S. Goldman. Waiting for coronary revascularization in Toronto: 2 years' experience with a regional referral office. *Canadian Medical Association Journal*, 149(7):955–962, 1993.

198. Ontario Ministry of Finance. Chapter 10: Immigration. In *Commission on the Reform of Ontario's Public Services*, pages 287–298, Queen's Printer for Ontario, 2012. http://www.fin.gov.on.ca/en/reformcommission/. Last accessed on April 11, 2019.

199. M. Chiu, P.C. Austin, D.G. Manuel, and Jack V. Tu. Cardiovascular risk factor profiles of recent immigrants vs long-term residents of Ontario: A multi-ethnic study. *Canadian Journal of Cardiology*, 28(1):20–26, 2011.

200. J. Chen, S.S. Rathore, M.J. Radford, Y. Wang, and H.M. Krumholz. Racial differences in the use of cardiac catheterization after acute myocardial infarction. *The New England Journal of Medicine*, 344(19):1443–1449, 2001.

201. K.M. King, N.A. Khan, and H. Quan. Ethnic variation in acute myocardial infarction presentation and access to care. *The American Journal of Cardiology*, 103(10):1368–1373, 2009.

202. N.A. Walton, D.K. Martin, E.H. Peter, D.M. Pringle, and P.A. Singer. Priority setting and cardiac surgery: A qualitative case study. *Health Policy*, 80:444–458, 2007.

203. M. Tenenhaus, V.E. Vinze, Y.M. Chatelin, and C. Lauro. PLS path modeling. *Computational Statistics and Data Analysis*, 48:159–205, 2005.

204. L. Schwartz, S. Woloshin, and J. Birkmeyer. How do elderly patients decide where to go for major surgery? Telephone interview survey. *BMJ*, 331:821, 2005.

205. L. Tao, J. Liu, and C.H.C. Leung. Adaptive operating room scheduling: An experimental study. In *Proceedings of the Second Advances in Health Informatics Conference, Toronto, Ontario, Canada*, pages 50–56, 2012.

206. H. Yong. *Applying Operations Research to Improve Resource Utilization in a Cardiac Surgical Service*. Thesis of Masters of Applied Science, University of Toronto, 2006.

207. F.J. Oeverdyk, S.C. Harvey, R.L. Fishman, and F. Shippey. Successful strategies for improving operating room efficiency at academic institutions. *Anesthesia and Analgesia*, 86(4):896–906, 1998.

208. E. Hans, G. Wullink, M.V. Houdenhoven, and G. Kazemier. Robust surgery loading. *European Journal of Operational Research*, 185(3):1038–1050, 2008.

209. I.M. Chakravarti, R.G. Laha, and J. Roy. *Handbook of Methods of Applied Statistics: Volume I*. John Wiley and Sons, 1967.

210. A. Clauset, C.R. Shalizi, and M.E.J. Newman. Power-law distributions in empirical data. *SIAM Review*, 51(4):661–703, 2009.

211. S. Kauffman. *At Home in the Universe: The Search for the Laws of Self-Organization and Complexity*. Oxford University Press, New York, 1995.

212. Cardiac Care Network of Ontario. Innovation: Annual report 08-09. 2009. http://www.ccn.on.ca/ccn_public/Uploadfiles/files/CCN_AnnualReport_2009(1).pdf. Last accessed on August 15, 2017.

213. Cardiac Care Network of Ontario. Cardiac care network: Annual report 09-10. 2010. http://www.ccn.on.ca/ccn_public/UploadFiles/files/CCN%20Annual%20Report%2009_10.pdf. Last accessed on August 15, 2017.

214. Cardiac Care Network of Ontario. Cardiac care network: Annual report 10-11. 2011. http://www.ccn.on.ca/ccn_public/Uploadfiles/files/CCN_Annual_Report_2011-_Final.pdf. Last accessed on August 15, 2017.

215. J.M. Kleinberg. Authoritative sources in a hyperlinked environment. *Journal of the ACM*, 46:604–632, 1999.

216. Cardiac Care Network of Ontario. Advanced adult cardiac care patient access management process: Better access to quality cardiac care. http://www.ccn.on.ca/ccn_public/uploadfiles/files/Patient%20Access%20Mgmnt%20diagram.pdf. Last accessed on August 15, 2017.

217. Ontario Ministry of Health and Long-Term Care. Ontario freezing doctor pay to invest in more community care for families and seniors. 2012. https://news.ontario.ca/mohltc/en/2012/05/ontario-freezing-doctor-pay-to-invest-in-more-community-care-for-families-and-seniors.html. Last accessed on April 11, 2019.

218. B. Chan. Access to physician services and patterns of practice. In *Cardiovascular Health and Services in Ontario: An ICES Atlas Toronto*, pages 301–318, D. Naylor, and P. Slaughter, eds., Institute for Clinical Evaluative Sciences, Ontario, 1999. https://www.ices.on.ca/Publications/Atlases-and-Reports/1999/Cardiovascular-health-and-services. Last accessed on April 11, 2019.

219. S.L. Grace, S.G. Witte, J. Brual, N. Suskin, L. Higginson, D. Alter, and D.E. Stewart. Contribution of patient and physician factors to cardiac rehabilitation referral: A prospective multilevel study. *Nature Clinical Practice Cardiovascular Medicine*, 5(10):653–662, 2008.

220. K.S. Kinchen, L.A. Cooper, D. Levine, N.Y. Wang, and N.R. Powe. Referral of patients to specialists: Factors affecting choice of specialist by primary care physicians. *Annals of Family Medicine*, 2(3):245–252, 2004.

221. L. Tao and J. Liu. An integrated analytical method for uncovering complex causal relationships in healthcare: A case study. In *Proceedings of the ACM SIGKDD Workshop on Health Informatics*, 2012.

222. Wakefield P.A., G.E. Randall, and G.M. Fiala. Competing for referrals for cardiac diagnostic tests: What do family physicians really want? *Journal of Medical Imaging and Radiation Sciences*, 43(3):155–160, 2012.

223. L. Kleinrock. *Queueing Systems: Volume I - Theory*. Wiley-Interscience, New York, 1975.

224. K.P. Burnham and D.R. Anderson. *Model selection and multi-model inference: A practical information-theoretic approach*. Springer, New York, 2002.

225. F. Moscone, E. Tosetti, and G. Vittadini. Social interaction in patients? hospital choice: Evidence from Italy. *Journal of the Royal Statistical Society: Series A (Statistics in Society)*, 175(2):453–472, 2012.

226. The Canadian Cardiovascular Society Workforce Project Steering Committee. Profile of the cardiovascular specialist physicians workforce in Canada. *Canadian Journal of Cardiology*, 18(8):835–852, 2002.

227. K. Jung, R. Feldman, and D. Scanlon. Where would you go for your next hospitalization? *Journal of Health Economics*, 30(4):832–841, 2011.

Notation Index

© Springer Nature Switzerland AG 2019

L. Tao, J. Liu, *Healthcare Service Management*, Health Information Science,
https://doi.org/10.1007/978-3-030-15385-4

Printed in the United States
By Bookmasters